Cases in
Human
Parasitology

Cases in Human Parasitology

Judith S. Heelan

Director of Microbiology
Memorial Hospital of Rhode Island
Pawtucket, Rhode Island
Associate Professor of Pathology and
Laboratory Medicine
Brown University
Providence, Rhode Island

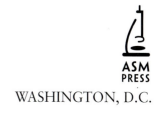

ASM
PRESS

WASHINGTON, D.C.

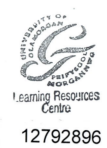

Address editorial correspondence to ASM Press, 1752 N St. NW,
Washington, DC 20036-2904, USA

Send orders to ASM Press, P.O. Box 605, Herndon, VA 20172, USA
Phone: (800) 546-2416 or (703) 661-1593
Fax: (703) 661-1501
E-mail: books@asmusa.org
Online: www.asmpress.org

Library of Congress Cataloging-in-Publication Data

Heelan, Judith Stephenson.
   Cases in human parasitology / Judith S. Heelan.
     p. ; cm.
 Includes bibliographical references and index.
 ISBN 1-55581-296-1 (pbk.)
 1. Parasitic diseases—Case studies.
 [DNLM: 1. Parasitic Diseases—diagnosis—Case Reports. 2. Para-
sites—microbiology—Case Reports. WC 695 H458c 2004] I. Title.

 RC119.H44 2004
 616.9′609—dc22

                                    2004004478

10 9 8 7 6 5 4 3 2 1

Cover and interior design: Susan Brown Schmidler

To my family, including my husband, Jack; my daughter, son-in-law,
and granddaughters, Stephanie, Brian, Emma, and Julia;
and my son and daughter-in-law, John and Beth;
and to the memory of my father, Francis J. Stephenson, whose support
and encouragement have always been my inspiration

Contents

Introduction

Parasites have been responsible for considerable morbidity and mortality throughout the ages worldwide, but today they are a problem mainly in developing countries. Although parasitic infections have a particularly strong impact on immunocompromised populations, many immunocompetent individuals also suffer from these illnesses.

Although some parasites are endemic to the United States, globalization has created considerable opportunities for infected travelers to bring back parasites from foreign countries. This book was written to provide examples of a variety of situations in which parasites are suspected of causing an infectious disease. In addition to infections caused by well-known parasites, as well as new and emerging parasites, *Cases in Human Parasitology* provides cases infrequently seen in this country to alert the reader that such uncommon infections may have been imported from elsewhere.

Previously written textbooks containing cases in microbiology and infectious diseases (P. H. Gilligan et al., *Cases in Medical Microbiology and Infectious Diseases* [American Society for Microbiology, Washington, D.C., 1992, 1997, 2003]) have proven to be successful in their efforts to provide an enjoyable and challenging educational tool for the reader. The purpose of *Cases in Human Parasitology* is to present cases solely involving parasites to supplement conventional textbooks in human parasitology and to provide an interesting and educational challenge to health care scientists. I was inspired to write the text for those individuals taking college or medical school courses in parasitology, for those being trained in hospitals in this field, and for those performing parasitology work in clinical laboratories, analyzing specimens to detect and identify parasites causing human disease.

The book is designed to stimulate discussion and to challenge students while emphasizing the relationship of diagnosis to patient care. It is hoped that the reader will learn to recognize the symptoms of parasitic diseases, to correlate the patient's history (travel, etc.) and symptoms to order laboratory procedures, and to guide treatment.

The book contains 62 cases of patients presenting to emergency departments or to their physicians with symptoms of a parasitic disease. The reader must develop a differential diagnosis and decide whether or not the patient is infected with a protozoan or helminth (worm). Most cases are accompanied by a color image(s) of the parasite causing the infection.

The book is divided into five sections, each dealing with a different group of parasites: intestinal protozoa (section I), blood and tissue protozoa (section II), cestodes, trematodes, and intestinal nematodes (section III), blood and tissue nematodes (section IV), and challenging cases (section V). The section entitled "Challenging Cases" covers nonparasitic infections in patients with symptoms closely resembling, and often confused with, those of parasitic infections.

At the beginning of each section is an introduction, which provides background information relating to the cases presented in that section. The introduction includes a brief discussion of parasites in that section, providing the reader with some clues to the etiology of those infections. Each case begins with the patient's history and symptoms. Travel history, residence, the age of the patient, seasonality, and eating habits are important in leading to the correct diagnosis and should be carefully noted. Relevant clinical findings and laboratory data are presented. The reader is asked to consider the differential diagnosis and is asked a number of questions about topics such as the following:

- the diagnosis of the illness
- the name of the parasite
- the life cycle of the parasite
- treatment, transmission, and prevention of the illness
- the epidemiology of the infection
- relevant clinical findings
- other parasites to consider in the differential diagnosis

Answers to the questions are provided at the end of each case presentation. A glossary and a list of figures are provided after section V.

The book may be used as an educational tool for educators in colleges and universities to reinforce didactic material taught in the classroom in courses in microbiology and parasitology in departments of microbiology or medical technology (clinical laboratory science); in hospital training programs in medical technology (clinical laboratory science); in programs in continuing medical education, to maintain the competence of clinical laboratory scientists doing parasitology work in clinical microbiology diagnostic laboratories and to satisfy regulatory requirements for various licensing boards; to train pathology residents and infectious disease fellows during their microbiology rotations, as well as to provide an educational tool for pathology residents preparing for board exams; and to teach first-year medical students taking courses in medical microbiology or infectious diseases and for medical students preparing for board exams. Many medical schools are currently using a case-based approach in their curriculum and have found that this method has been proven to be effective in other areas of medicine.

Acknowledgments

I thank members of the editorial staff of ASM Press for their assistance and patience during the preparation of this book. I also thank the reviewers for their comments and suggestions for improvements to the text.

Many of the illustrations were produced with the assistance of Stanley Schwartz of the Department of Pathology at the Memorial Hospital of Rhode Island. I thank him for his help. These images would not have been possible without his expertise.

This section is intended to introduce the reader to the usefulness of patient symptoms and history, as well as laboratory findings, in the diagnosis of infection with an intestinal protozoan. Pathogenic intestinal protozoa discussed in this section include amebae, flagellates, ciliates, coccidia, and microsporidia.

Human infection with amebae, which move by means of pseudopods and are classified in the subphylum Sarcodina of the phylum Sarcomastigophora, is called amebiasis. *Entamoeba histolytica,* which may cause amebic dysentery, is the most pathogenic of the intestinal amebae and may cause extraintestinal infections, especially liver abscesses, as well as gastrointestinal disease. It must be distinguished from nonpathogenic amebae that may be infecting the patient.

Although *Blastocystis hominis* is of uncertain taxonomic affiliation, having previously been classified as a yeast, it is currently considered to be a protozoan. When this parasite is present in the absence of other pathogens, it is likely to be the cause of gastrointestinal symptoms.

Intestinal flagellates, which are members of the subphylum Mastigophora of the phylum Sarcomastigophora, move by means of whiplike appendages known as flagella. *Giardia lamblia* is the most common of all intestinal flagellates and is responsible for most cases of gastrointestinal infection. *Dientamoeba fragilis,* originally classified as an ameba, is now considered to be a flagellate and is thought to be responsible for some cases of gastrointestinal disease.

The only pathogenic ciliate, in the phylum Ciliophora, is *Balantidium coli,* the largest protozoan parasite known to cause gastrointestinal infections in humans. Pigs act as reservoirs of infection for this uncommon parasite.

The traditional method used to diagnose amebiasis, giardiasis, or balantidiasis is the routine microscopic examination for the presence of characteristic trophozoites and cysts of the parasite in stained and unstained preparations of fecal specimens. It is imperative that microscopic preparations be examined by experienced and well-trained medical technologists (clinical laboratory scientists). Specimens must be collected properly and should be brought immediately to the laboratory or placed in fixatives. A minimum of three specimens should be collected over a period of 10 days. More sensitive diagnostic techniques have recently been developed to detect parasites in fecal specimens, but these assays are not always available in clinical laboratories.

Coccidia are nonmotile, obligate intracellular parasites with complex life cycles; they are found in a variety of animals, and some species are able to cause human infection, particularly in immunocompromised hosts. *Cryptosporidium parvum* causes self-limited diarrhea in immunocompetent individuals but often causes intractable diarrhea in immunocompromised hosts, especially in AIDS patients.

Isospora belli also causes diarrhea in AIDS patients but is less common than *Cryptosporidium parvum*. *Cyclospora cayetanensis* is another member of the coccidia that is well recognized to be a cause of diarrhea in both immunocompetent and immunocompromised individuals.

Special studies, including the modified acid-fast procedure, may be necessary to diagnose infections caused by these protozoa. Careful determination of size and shape allows differentiation of these parasites.

Microsporidia cause opportunistic infections in immunocompromised individuals. They produce tiny spores, which are difficult to detect. Methods of detection include electron microscopic examination of tissue specimens, histological techniques, and a modification of the trichrome stain.

Most patients infected with intestinal protozoa present with gastrointestinal symptoms, especially diarrhea. These symptoms may also be due to a variety of other microorganisms or may result from noninfectious causes. Microorganisms which may cause gastrointestinal symptoms include viruses, bacteria, and fungi, as well as parasites.

A careful history is important in making an accurate diagnosis of an intestinal protozoan infection. Travel history is particularly relevant, since many of these parasites are found only in certain geographical areas. Increased travel has led to a global approach to the diagnosis of parasitic infections. Other significant findings include the age of the patient and attendance at school or, especially, day care centers, where person-to-person transmission of infection among young children is more likely to occur, often resulting in outbreaks of disease.

Most gastrointestinal pathogens are spread by the oral-fecal route. Parasites may be ingested from contaminated food or water or from contaminated inanimate objects, especially by children. Food may be infected in a variety of ways. Sick food handlers may also be responsible for the contamination. Poor sanitary conditions and the absence of good hygiene practices provide mechanisms for transmission of parasites. Proper purification of drinking water is essential, as is the protection of water supplies from reservoir hosts infected with parasites, since contamination of the water by animals may occur.

A number of drugs are available to treat patients infected with pathogenic intestinal protozoa.

Case 1

A 22-year-old male college student, who had recently returned from a surfing trip to Acapulco, Mexico, presented to the emergency department suffering from crampy abdominal pain, malaise, nausea, fever, and bloody, mucoid diarrhea. Stool specimens were collected and sent to the laboratory for routine culture for enteric bacilli and examination for ova and parasites.

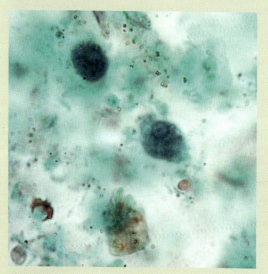

Stool cultures were negative for bacterial pathogens. A moderate number of ameboid trophozoites, measuring 20 to 30 μm, with finely granular cytoplasm, evenly distributed peripheral nuclear chromatin, and ingested red blood cells were seen in the permanent trichrome stain. A characteristic trophozoite is shown in Fig. 1.1. No cyst forms were seen.

Figure 1.1

QUESTIONS

1. Based on the morphological description given, which intestinal parasite would you suspect is causing this patient's infection? Could this parasite be confused with nonpathogenic parasites? If so, which nonpathogenic parasites could it be confused with?

2. Although no information regarding the stool consistency (formed, semisolid, or liquid) was given, what would you suspect the consistency of this patient's stool to be? Why?

3. Which nonpathogenic parasite is morphologically indistinguishable from this parasite? What characteristic can be used to differentiate pathogenic from nonpathogenic species of this parasite?

4. Is this parasite capable of causing extraintestinal infection? Explain.

5. How is this parasite transmitted?

6. What laboratory techniques are recommended to diagnose infection with this parasite?

7. Should this patient be treated? How?

8. Discuss the pathogenesis of amebiasis.

9. Describe the life cycle of this parasite.

10. Discuss the epidemiology of this infection.

11. Discuss the prevention and control of amebiasis.

ANSWERS

1. The description of the parasite most closely resembles the intestinal ameba *Entamoeba histolytica*. This parasite causes amebic dysentery with symptoms as described in this patient, including bloody diarrhea, slight fever, abdominal pain, nausea, and malaise. Nonpathogenic amebae which may be confused with *E. histolytica* include *Entamoeba coli*, which has a similar size, although the cysts of *Entamoeba coli* contain as many as 8 nuclei (possibly 16) when mature as opposed to a maximum of 4 nuclei in *E. histolytica*.

   The trophozoites and cysts of *Entamoeba hartmanni* are identical to those of *E. histolytica* but are smaller. The trophozoite of this ameba measures 5 to 12 μm, and the cyst measures 5 to 10 μm. This parasite was once known as "small-race *E. histolytica*." The trophozoites of *Entamoeba dispar*, a separate species once considered to be a strain of *E. histolytica*, do not ingest red blood cells.

2. The stool specimen was probably liquid, since trophozoites were present but no cyst forms were observed. In liquid stool, amebic trophozoites predominate, while formed stools contain primarily the cyst form. In semiformed specimens, both trophozoites and cysts are usually seen.

3. It is now recognized that clinical isolates of *E. histolytica* may be divided into pathogenic and nonpathogenic species, called *E. histolytica* and *E. dispar*, respectively. The two otherwise morphologically indistinguishable species may be differentiated by isoenzyme analysis (zymodemes), which is not usually available in most clinical laboratories. It has been suggested that only parasites with certain isoenzyme patterns are capable of causing disease. As stated above, only invasive *E. histolytica*, unlike the noninvasive *E. dispar*, ingests red blood cells.

4. Yes, *E. histolytica* is capable of causing extraintestinal infection. It is the only ameba capable of causing infection at sites outside of the intestine. Trophozoites may invade the wall of the colon and enter the blood circulation, thereby spreading to other areas of the body, including the lungs, spleen and brain, resulting in the development of extraintestinal abscesses.

5. *E. histolytica* is mostly transmitted person to person by means of fecally contaminated food and water containing amebic cysts, although sexual transmission has been reported. After ingestion, excystation occurs with formation of four trophozoites. Asymptomatic carriers are of great importance in the transmission of disease, since they generally produce only cysts, which are more resistant to destruction than are the trophozoites produced by patients with acute forms of amebiasis. Trophozoites do not survive very long, outside the body of the host.

6. The laboratory diagnosis of amebiasis is usually made by examination of fecal specimens for the presence of typical trophozoites and cysts of *E. histolytica*. Successful diagnosis is dependent on collection of proper specimens and examination by well-trained and experienced laboratory personnel. Direct saline wet preparations may be useful in detecting motile trophozoites, especially in liquid stool specimens, and concentration techniques may allow the observation of amebic cysts. However, the permanent stained smear, such as the trichrome or iron hematoxylin

stain, is most useful in the identification of amebic trophozoites and cysts. A permanent stained smear should be made on all stool specimens, regardless of the consistency of the specimen. A minimum of three specimens should be collected over a period of 10 days. As mentioned above, microscopic methods do not always allow differentiation of the pathogenic species of *E. histolytica* from the nonpathogenic *E. dispar.* Typical trophozoites which do not contain ingested red blood cells should be reported as *E. histolytica/E. dispar* group.

Serological procedures are of limited value for intestinal disease. The enzyme immunoassay has been reported to detect specific antibody in about 70% of patients with active intestinal infection. Procedures for detecting amebic antibodies are more successful in the diagnosis of systemic infections. Methods include the indirect hemagglutination assay, the enzyme-linked immunosorbent assay (ELISA) with microtiter plates, and the indirect immunofluorescence assay (IFA).

Commercial immunoassay kits used to detect amebic antigens in stool specimens, including a combination kit for the detection of *Giardia lamblia* and *E. histolytica,* are also available. An immunochromatographic lateral-flow membrane assay, using a cartridge format, is a sensitive, specific, rapid, easy-to-read immunoassay for the diagnosis of amebiasis. This method relies on capillary action, since amebic antigens are captured by specific antibody as the sample moves laterally through the unit. Although most fecal immunoassays fail to distinguish the nonpathogenic *E. dispar* from the pathogenic *E. histolytica,* one commercially available kit does distinguish between the two parasites. This assay may have limited use, since fresh or frozen stool is required for testing and many laboratories receive their specimens in preservatives.

A closed-tube real-time PCR method has been developed to distinguish *E. histolytica* from *E. dispar* directly from feces. This method appears to be highly sensitive and specific but requires the presence of a LightCycler.

7. Except for asymptomatic cyst passage, when a luminal drug may be sufficient, all patients diagnosed with *E. histolytica* infection should be treated with both metronidazole and a luminal amebicide such as iodoquinol or diloxanide furoate.

8. Patients with amebiasis usually experience abdominal pain and bloody diarrhea, although asymptomatic carriers may exist. In patients with amebic dysentery, ulcers may form in the appendix, cecum, and other parts of the colon. Ulcers are usually flask-shaped and appear raised, with small mucosal openings. An eroded area lies beneath the surface of the ulcer. Symptoms of amebic dysentery often resemble those of ulcerative colitis or diverticulitis.

9. The life cycles of nonpathogenic amebae are similar to that of *E. histolytica,* except for the invasive stage resulting in extraintestinal infection. The infection begins when mature cysts (the infective stage) are ingested. The mature cyst passes through the stomach and excysts in the lower ileum of the small intestine. Here the cyst develops into the trophozoite form and multiplies by binary fission. Trophozoites continue to reproduce in the lumen of the colon. They may encyst. Immature cysts (with one or two nuclei) are passed in the feces, although cysts may develop to maturity (with four nuclei) before being excreted. Trophozoites, immature cysts, and mature cysts may be found in the feces, although trophozoites are usually found

only in liquid feces. As mentioned above, trophozoites of E. *histolytica* may invade the wall of the colon, multiply, and pass into the circulation, causing extraintestinal infection.

10. Although amebiasis is found worldwide, E. *histolytica* is most prevalent and more severe in tropical and subtropical locations. Asymptomatic infections occur more commonly in temperate climates. Dietary deficiencies may play a role in the severity of disease. Crowded conditions, such as those found in orphanages, prisons, and mental institutions, may exacerbate the transmission of disease. In the United States, amebiasis is more prevalent in rural areas, especially in the southeastern and southwestern parts of the country, and among lower socioeconomic groups.

11. Prevention and control of amebiasis lie in the destruction of the hardy cysts of E. *histolytica,* which are usually transmitted in water. A combination of filtration and chemical treatment is required to provide a parasite-free water supply, since the amebae are resistant to chlorination alone. Tourists in areas of endemic infection should avoid drinking local water and using ice, which may have been made from contaminated water. Fruits and vegetables should be washed in boiled or treated water before being eaten. Adequate disposal of human waste is imperative, and the practice of using human feces (night soil) as fertilizer should be discouraged. Contamination of food by insects, especially flies and cockroaches, should be prevented.

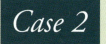

Case 2

A 25-year-old woman had recently returned from a trip to the Rocky Mountains. She had been traveling with a group of campers, who had obtained their drinking water from a lake. A few days after returning home, she presented to her internist suffering from profuse watery diarrhea, crampy epigastric pain, and foul-smelling flatulence. She discovered that most of the other campers had reported symptoms similar to her own.

Three stool specimens were submitted for laboratory analysis. All specimens were negative for enteric bacterial pathogens, and two were also negative for parasites. Since the specimens for ova and parasites were received in vials containing the preservatives polyvinyl alcohol and 10% formalin, no wet mounts were made to detect motility. A permanent trichrome stain revealed rare, oval protozoan trophozoites, measuring 9 to 20 µm in length and 5 to 15 µm in width. The broad anterior end of each trophozoite contained a concave area which covered half the ventral surface. The structure of this parasite gave the overall appearance of a "smiling face" (Fig. 2.1). Rare cysts, having four nuclei, and characteristic median bodies and longitudinal fibers were also seen. Typical cysts are demonstrated in Fig. 2.2.

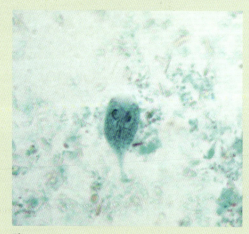

Figure 2.1

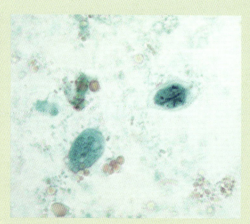

Figure 2.2

QUESTIONS

1. Which protozoan parasite is causing the camper's infection? Which form of this parasite is infectious?

2. How is this parasite transmitted?

3. How can this infection be controlled and prevented?

4. How does this parasite attach itself to the intestinal wall? Which condition might result as a consequence of this attachment?

5. How is this infection treated?

6. Describe the life cycle of this parasite.

7. Describe the pathogenesis of this infection.

8. How is the laboratory diagnosis of this infection made?

9. Discuss the epidemiology of this infection.

10. How does the structure of these trophozoites account for the "smiling-face" appearance?

ANSWERS

1. The protozoan parasite causing the camper's infection is *Giardia lamblia* (also called *G. intestinalis* or *G. duodenalis*). The cyst form of this parasite is infectious.

2. Transmission of *G. lamblia* usually occurs by the fecal-oral route from ingestion of cysts in contaminated water. Many water sources, such as ponds, lakes, and streams, harbor these cysts as a result of fecal contamination by animals or humans. Although foods are less likely to serve as vehicles of infection, contaminated fruits and raw vegetables may transmit disease. Person-to-person transmission through oral or anal sexual practices may also occur.

3. Giardiasis may be prevented by drinking only treated water. Filtration must be part of the water purification process to remove the cysts of *G. lamblia* from drinking water because the parasite is resistant to chlorine. Water should therefore be treated by filtration techniques in addition to chlorination. Halazone tablets are frequently used for this purpose. Another preventive measure is the protection of water supplies from reservoir hosts, such as beavers and muskrats. Safe sexual practices should prevent sexual transmission of this parasite.

4. The ventral side of *G. lamblia* is covered by a sucking disk. The parasite attaches to the mucosa of the small intestine by means of this structure. The firm attachment to the mucosa interferes with dislodgement during intestinal peristalsis. Malabsorption may result when the parasite mechanically interferes with intestinal absorption. Certain intestinal mucosal enzymes may also be inhibited. Structural changes in intestinal villi are also thought to be responsible for the malabsorption syndrome.

5. The treatment of choice for giardiasis is metronidazole. Alternate choices include quinacrine, paromomycin, tinidazole, and furazolidone. It is recommended that all patients with giardiasis, asymptomatic as well as symptomatic, be treated, because subclinical malabsorption may occur and because asymptomatic carriers may pose risks for the spread of infection.

6. The cyst is the infective stage of *G. lamblia* and is acquired by ingestion of contaminated water or food. After leaving the stomach, the cyst passes into the small intestine. Excystation usually occurs in the crypts of the duodenum. Approximately every 8 h, the parasite multiplies by longitudinal binary fission, with the production of two trophozoites. Trophozoites attach to the mucosa of the duodenum by using their sucking disks. Encystation occurs when the trophozoites enter the large intestine. Trophozoites and cysts, which are diagnostic for giardiasis, may be found in the feces. The predominant form in the feces is usually the cyst, since the trophozoites are highly susceptible to environmental conditions outside of the body.

7. Symptoms of giardiasis usually develop after an incubation period of approximately 2 to 3 weeks and may mimic food poisoning, amebiasis, or bacillary dysentery. These symptoms include nausea, explosive watery foul-smelling diarrhea, abdominal discomfort, flatulence, and anorexia. The patient often describes having a rotten-egg taste in his or her mouth. Fat-soluble vitamin deficiencies and folic acid deficiencies may occur. Hypogammaglobulinemia and structural changes in intestinal villi may develop. In severe cases, the malabsorption syndrome may lead to steatorrhea. Patients may also be asymptomatic.

8. *G. lamblia* may be detected by routine examinations for ova and parasites; however, the parasite is easily missed, even when multiple stool specimens are examined. The concentration technique may be useful in detecting trophozoites or cysts of this parasite; however, the permanent stained smear, using the trichrome or iron hematoxylin stain, is more valuable in making the diagnosis. As with the amebae, liquid or soft fecal specimens from infected patients are more apt to contain actively motile trophozoites while cysts are more likely to be found in formed stools. The presence of either trophozoites or cysts is diagnostic for infection.

Duodenal aspirates may also be examined for the presence of the parasite. The Entero-Test capsule may be used as a noninvasive method to sample duodenal contents. A weighted length of nylon yarn is coiled within a gelatin capsule. One end of the yarn is taped to the patient's cheek. After being swallowed, the capsule dissolves and the yarn passes into the duodenum. After 4 to 6 h of incubation, the line is retrieved and material adhering to it is removed by pressing the yarn between the thumb and the forefinger of a gloved hand onto a glass slide, coverslipped, and examined under the microscope.

Although procedures exist for the cultivation of this protozoan parasite in vitro, these methods are labor-intensive, difficult, and expensive and are not useful in the clinical diagnostic laboratory; they are used primarily as research tools rather than diagnostic tools.

Serological assays for antibody to *G. lamblia* usually lack sensitivity. Antigen detection methods have been more successful in diagnosing giardiasis. Immunofluorescence assay methods and enzyme immunoassays using microtiter plates are commercially available for the detection of *G. lamblia* antigen in stool specimens. Some of these tests have shown sensitivities and specificities comparable to or better than those of microscopic examination for cysts or trophozoites. Immunochromatographic lateral-flow membrane assays, using a cartridge format, are sensitive, specific, rapid, and easy-to-read immunoassays for the diagnosis of giardiasis. This method relies on capillary action, since parasite antigens are captured by specific antibody as the sample moves laterally through the unit. Combination kits to detect *G. lamblia* and *Cryptosporidium parvum* are commercially available.

9. Found worldwide, *G. lamblia* is probably the most common intestinal parasite in the United States, with the exception of *Blastocystis hominis*. It resides in the gastrointestinal tract of a variety of mammals, including humans. Many water sources, such as ponds, lakes, and streams, contain *G. lamblia* cysts due to fecal contamination by humans or animals. This infection is more prevalent in day care settings and nursery schools, where young children are apt to gather in close contact with each other. Patients who have had gastrectomies, with the resulting absence of gastric acidity, are more likely to acquire this infection. There is also an increased prevalence of giardiasis among homosexual men, most probably due to anal and/or oral sexual practices.

10. The trophozoite of *G. lamblia* has two nuclei ("eyes"), which are laterally located in the bilaterally symmetrical trophozoite. Each nucleus contains a large, central karyosome ("eyeball"). An axostyle ("nose"), consisting of two axonemes, divides the flagellate into two halves. Two curved median or parabasal bodies ("mouth") cross the axoneme at an oblique angle. Overall, these features give the trophozoite the appearance of a smiling face.

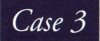

A previously healthy 32-year-old woman with a history of several weeks of diarrhea alternating with constipation, abdominal discomfort, vomiting, anorexia, intense fatigue, myalgia, and other "flu-like" symptoms went to her internist for treatment. Stool specimens were collected and submitted to the laboratory for routine bacterial culture as well as examination for ova and parasites.

The patient had not traveled outside the United States but remarked that her symptoms had developed a few days after she attended a June wedding in Florida. She had been told that several other guests at the wedding had developed similar symptoms. When the routine tests for enteric pathogens were reported as being negative, the physician ordered special tests, including special stains for coccidia. Microscopic examination of a modified acid-fast-stained smear revealed spherical structures approximately 8 to 10 μm in diameter, showing a range of intensity from colorless to dark red (Fig. 3.1). The spherical structures showed autofluorescence when viewed using a UV microscope.

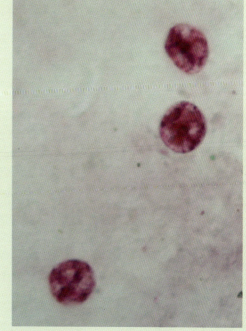

Figure 3.1

QUESTIONS

1. Which intestinal protozoan parasite might be causing this patient's symptoms? Explain your answer based on the results of laboratory tests.

2. List two other protozoan parasites which might be confused with this parasite. How may these three parasites be distinguished from each other?

3. How does this patient's history correlate with this diagnosis?

4. Where have outbreaks of this infection occurred?

5. Does this parasite cause more serious illness in immunocompromised individuals?

6. Should the patient be treated? If so, how?

7. How can this infection be controlled and prevented?

ANSWERS

1. *Cyclospora cayetanensis* is the probable cause of this patient's infection. The nonrefractile, wrinkled oocysts of this parasite would probably not be seen on routine stool examination. The modified acid-fast stain demonstrates oocysts ranging in intensity from unstained glassy, wrinkled spheres to light pink or dark red structures. UV epifluorescence techniques used to detect autofluorescence show a weak 1+ to 2+ green or blue fluorescence. When the formalin/ethyl acetate concentration procedure is used, centrifugation should be performed at $500 \times g$ for 10 min. Although electron microscopy may be used as a research tool, it is not likely to be helpful in making a diagnosis of infection with *C. cayetanensis*.

2. *Cryptosporidium parvum* and *Isospora belli* may resemble *Cyclospora cayetanensis* in that they both stain pink with the modified acid-fast stain. However, the marked difference in size and shape allows them to be differentiated from each other. The oocysts of *Cryptosporidium parvum* are smaller (4 to 6 μm) than those of *Cyclospora cayetanensis* (8 to 10 μm), whereas those of *I. belli* are larger (25 to 30 μm). *Cryptosporidium parvum*, unlike *Cyclospora cayetanensis* and *I. belli*, does not autofluoresce under UV light. *I. belli* not only is larger than *Cryptosporidium parvum* and *Cyclospora cayetanensis* but also is more ellipsoidal. It is important to carefully measure all acid-fast oocysts, especially if they appear to be about twice the size of *Cryptosporidium* oocysts.

3. *Cyclospora cayetanensis* is usually transmitted in contaminated food. Infections resulting from ingestion of contaminated fruits, such as imported strawberries and raspberries, have been reported. In this case, the fact that several guests from the wedding developed gastrointestinal symptoms is strongly suggestive of a food-associated infection.

4. The distribution of this parasite is worldwide, including the United States, Canada, the Caribbean, Central and South America, Southeast Asia, Eastern Europe, Australia, Haiti, and Nepal. Cases in the United States are usually associated with travelers returning from developing nations. Outbreaks of cyclosporiasis in the United States have been reported in 20 states, including Florida, Illinois, California, and New York. There is an increased risk of developing cyclosporiasis in late spring and summer; this is thought to be associated with heavy rains during these seasons, such as the monsoon season in Nepal.

5. Although most outbreak cases of cyclosporiasis have been found in immunocompetent individuals, immunocompromised individuals, particularly AIDS patients, are more likely to suffer from long-lasting cyclosporiasis, with symptoms continuing for many weeks or months. Relapses are common; periods of diarrhea often alternate with periods of constipation. Biliary disease has also been found in this group of patients.

6. Unlike cryptosporidiosis, treatment is available for cyclosporiasis. Symptomatic patients may be treated with trimethoprim-sulfamethoxazole, which is the drug of choice, although relapses are common.

7. Good hygiene practices, as well as proper water treatment methods, are imperative in controlling infection with *C. cayetanensis*. In areas of endemic infection, water should be boiled before being consumed. Thorough washing of fruits and vegetables, particularly those imported from other countries, reduces the likelihood of contamination of these food items.

Case 4

A 25-year-old American homosexual man was seen in the emergency room for bloody diarrhea and crampy abdominal pain of several weeks' duration and was treated based on the results of laboratory studies. His symptoms resolved, and he appeared to make a full recovery.

Six months later, he presented to his family physician suffering from weight loss, malaise, fever, fatigue, and abdominal pain in the right upper quadrant. Laboratory studies revealed leukocytosis, mild anemia, and elevated levels of liver enzymes, including alkaline phosphatase and transaminases. Stool specimens for culture and examination for ova and parasites were negative for bacterial pathogens and parasites.

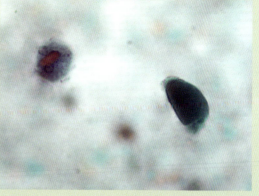

Figure 4.1

A computed tomography (CT) scan of the liver was performed and revealed several hepatic lesions. Because of the CT scan abnormalities, an ELISA for serum antibodies was ordered, which confirmed the diagnosis of his illness. A cyst of the parasite causing his illness is shown in Fig. 4.1.

QUESTIONS

1. What is this patient's diagnosis? Which protozoan parasite is shown in Fig. 4.1?

2. How does the patient's illness correlate with his previous episode of bloody diarrhea? Why is the patient's stool specimen negative for parasites?

3. Describe the life cycle of this parasite as it relates to this patient's infection.

4. Can abscesses caused by this parasite occur in organs other than the liver?

5. Which laboratory tests were probably used to make a diagnosis at the time the patient was first seen in the emergency room? Which specimen might prove useful in making a diagnosis during the patient's latest visit?

6. What risk to the patient exists in performance of a surgical procedure to obtain a liver aspirate?

7. How might the patient's homosexuality be related to his infection?

8. How should this patient be treated?

9. Which serological tests were probably ordered to confirm the diagnosis?

10. Discuss methods of control and prevention of infection with this parasite.

ANSWERS

1. The diagnosis of this patient's illness is a liver abscess, probably caused by the protozoan parasite *Entamoeba histolytica*.

2. The patient had been treated 6 months earlier, based on "results of laboratory studies," for bloody diarrhea, which was most probably a case of amebiasis (or amebic dysentery) caused by *E. histolytica*. The "laboratory study" was probably an examination for ova and parasites. Although some patients diagnosed with amebic liver abscesses have concurrent amebic colitis, they usually have no bowel symptoms, and stool specimens are negative for *E. histolytica* cysts and trophozoites when a routine examination for ova and parasites is performed.

3. The infection begins when mature cysts (the infective stage) of *E. histolytica* are ingested. The mature cyst passes through the stomach and excysts in the lower ileum of the small intestine. Here, the cyst develops into the trophozoite form and multiplies by binary fission. The trophozoites continue to multiply and may encyst in the lumen of the large intestine. Immature cysts (with one or two nuclei) are passed in the feces, although cysts may develop to maturity (with four nuclei) before being excreted. Trophozoites, immature cysts, and mature cysts may be found in the feces, although trophozoites are usually found only in liquid feces.

Extraintestinal infection with *E. histolytica* occurs when amebic trophozoites invade the wall of the colon and enter the blood circulation, thereby spreading to other areas of the body.

4. Abscesses caused by *E. histolytica* may occur in the lungs, spleen, and the brain, although liver abscesses are most common.

5. A routine stool examination for ova and parasites probably revealed the characteristic trophozoites and/or cysts of *E. histolytica*. These trophozoites, measuring 12 to 60 μm, have finely granular cytoplasm and evenly distributed peripheral nuclear chromatin and frequently reveal ingested red blood cells. Cyst forms measure 10 to 20 μm and contain four nuclei plus cigar-shaped structures (chromatoid bodies) with smooth, rounded, blunt ends. As mentioned above, this test is negative in most patients with amebic abscesses.

Aspirates obtained from liver abscesses may be examined for amebic parasites. However, amebae are usually present only in the last portion of aspirated material, from the hepatic tissue of the abscess wall, and not from necrotic material from the center of the abscess. The positive yield from liver aspirates, however, is low, even when the specimen is collected under optimal conditions. The diagnosis of these abscesses is usually confirmed serologically.

Although procedures exist for the cultivation of this protozoan parasite in vitro, these methods are labor-intensive, difficult, and expensive and are not useful in the clinical diagnostic laboratory; they are used primarily as research tools rather than diagnostic tools.

6. A liver abscess resembles a hydatid cyst, which develops as a result of infection with a tapeworm in the genus *Echinococcus*. In a surgical procedure to obtain an aspirate from what is thought to be a liver abscess but is actually a hydatid cyst, there is a risk of anaphylaxis, an allergic reaction which may result in shock and death, and the possibility of spread of the echinococcal infection by seeding the peritoneal cavity with material from the hydatid cyst, which is known as hydatid sand. CT scans are recommended to detect liver abscesses.

7. In the 1960s, social changes influencing homosexual behavior contributed to the increase in the number of sexually transmitted diseases, including infection with *E. histolytica*. Sexual transmission of amebiasis occurred mainly among urban homosexual men. *E. histolytica* was, at that time, considered to be one of the most common pathogens included among the sexually transmitted microorganisms causing what is known as the "gay bowel syndrome" in homosexual men.

The fact that many homosexual men found to be positive for *E. histolytica* were asymptomatic was initially a cause for concern. This is because asymptomatic carriers are of great importance in the transmission of disease, since they generally produce only cysts, which are more resistant to destruction than are the trophozoites produced by patients with acute forms of amebiasis. However, recent evidence suggests that the parasite identified in many of these asymptomatic individuals (referred to as the *E. histolytica/E. dispar* group) may actually have been the nonpathogenic *E. dispar* and that the incidence of infection with the pathogenic *E. histolytica* is much lower than it was thought to be.

8. Patients with hepatic disease should be treated with metronidazole plus one of the luminal drugs, such as iodoquinol or diloxanide furoate.

9. Positive serological tests are useful to support clinical findings in these cases. Serological assays including the ELISA technique, indirect hemagglutination, and the IFA, were probably ordered to confirm the diagnosis of amebiasis in this patient.

10. Control and prevention of amebiasis lie in the ability to destroy the hardy cysts of *E. histolytica*, which are usually transmitted in water. A combination of filtration and chemical treatment is recommended to destroy the parasite. Although relatively resistant, cysts are usually killed by drying, by temperatures higher than 55°C, by superchlorination, or by the addition of iodide to drinking water. Local water and ice made from local water sources in areas of endemic infection should be avoided. Fruits and vegetables in such areas should be washed before being consumed. Adequate disposal of human waste is essential.

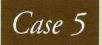

Case 5

A 29-year-old human immunodeficiency virus (HIV)-infected man presented to his primary-care doctor complaining of chronic, severe, profuse, nonbloody, watery diarrhea. He had nausea and a poor appetite and had experienced a 15-lb weight loss over the past several months. His laboratory test results included a very low CD4 lymphocyte count (of only 100). Stool specimens cultured for enteric bacilli were negative. Fecal specimens examined for ova and parasites, which included a microscopic study of the concentrated sediment and a permanent trichrome-stained smear, were negative for intestinal parasites.

A special stain was then ordered in the microbiology laboratory, which led to a diagnosis of intestinal parasites. Microscopic examination revealed very tiny parasites, not much larger than staphylococcal cells. A typical parasite is shown in Fig. 5.1.

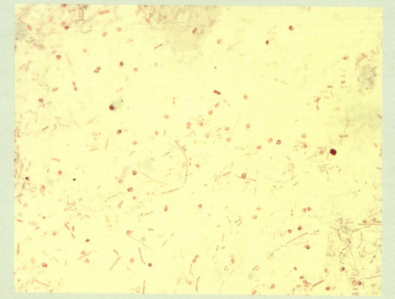

Figure 5.1

QUESTIONS

1. Which stain was used to stain the parasite shown in Fig. 5.1?

2. Which group of obligate intracellular protozoan parasites would you suspect of causing this infection in an AIDS patient? Which member of this group would you expect might be causing this patient's infection? Why?

3. How do these parasites differ from other intracellular intestinal protozoans?

4. How do these parasites multiply?

5. How is infection with this parasite transmitted?

6. How is the laboratory diagnosis of infection with this parasite made?

ANSWERS

1. The parasite was stained by the chromotrope stain method (see the answer to question 6).

2. The obligate intracellular protozoan parasite was probably a member of the phylum Microspora. These parasites have increasingly been recognized as opportunistic pathogens in patients with AIDS. The microorganism was probably either *Enterocytozoon bieneusi* or *Encephalitozoon intestinalis,* which are species of microsporidia frequently isolated from AIDS patients with diarrhea. Infections with *Encephalitozoon intestinalis,* unlike infections with *Enterocytozoon bieneusi,* may respond to treatment with albendazole.

3. The microsporidia are distinguished from other intracellular intestinal protozoans by the production of characteristic environmentally resistant spores, measuring 1 to 5 μm, each of which contains a coiled, tubular extrusion apparatus (polar tubule or filament). The polar tubule is extruded forcefully when contact is made with adjacent host cells. It penetrates a host cell, and the contents of the spore are then injected into the cytoplasm of the host cell.

4. After introduction of the infectious material (sporoplasm) into the host cell, extensive multiplication of the microsporidia takes place in the cytoplasm of the host cells in the small intestine. Cell division occurs by the processes of binary fission (merogony), multiple fission (schizogony), and spore production (sporogony). During sporogony, a thick spore wall forms, which provides protection against harmful environmental effects.

5. Spores of microsporidia disseminate within host tissues or are released into the lumen of the intestine and are passed in the feces. The spores are environmentally resistant and may be ingested by other humans. Although most cases of microsporidiosis occur in AIDS patients, cases have occurred in patients with healthy immune systems.

6. The diagnosis of infection with *Enterocytozoon bieneusi, Encephalitozoon intestinalis,* and other microsporidia is difficult due to the small size (1.5 to 3 μm) of the spores, which may be overlooked by workers using routine laboratory procedures. Spores may be identified in biopsy material by use of the Giemsa stain and the histological periodic acid-Schiff stain.

A smear of fecal specimens may also be stained by the chromotrope Gram method or by the modified trichrome stain, in which the chromotrope 2R is 10 times more concentrated than it is in the routine trichrome stain for stool. To enhance the ability to make a diagnosis using this method, the stool smear must be very thin. Several formulations of this stain, including the Weber green stain, using a fast green counterstain, and the Ryan blue modified trichrome stain, using an aniline blue counterstain, are commercially available. In both methods, spores stain pinkish-red with clear central or polar zones, making the stained areas appear as bands. This is a characteristic finding for the identification of microsporidia. Since the penetration of the stain into the spore wall is difficult, the staining time is much longer than in the traditional trichrome stain method. Microscopic examination should be done at a magnification of ×1,000 or higher. However, heating the stain to 50°C both decreases the staining time and greatly increases the quality of the stain. Chemofluorescent (optical brightening) agents are useful in the detection of the spores of microsporidia. Using Calcofluor White, the spores may be seen using a fluorescence microscope. These agents, although sensitive for the detection of microsporidia, are not specific for these organisms.

Although procedures exist for the cultivation of this protozoan parasite in vitro, they are labor-intensive, difficult, and expensive and are not useful in the clinical diagnostic laboratory. Destruction of the parasite in the presence of other micro-organisms, such as adenovirus, in the fecal specimens is also a problem. These methods are used primarily as research tools rather than diagnostic tools.

Although PCR methods have been used for the detection of microsporidia, these methods have been developed for use in research laboratories and are not generally suitable for use in the routine clinical laboratory. A real-time PCR method has been developed for the detection of *Encephalitozoon intestinalis* from liquid stool specimens. This assay, using a LightCycler apparatus, appears to be more user-friendly and more suitable for use in the clinical laboratory.

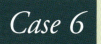

Case 6 A 39-year-old HIV-infected patient presented to his primary-care doctor reporting severe diarrhea of several months' duration. He was not receiving antiretroviral therapy, due to severe side effects of the drugs. His diarrhea was watery and profuse, with no sign of blood. The patient showed signs of dehydration, probably due to massive fluid loss. Nonprescription antidiarrheal medications, such as loperamide HCl (Imodium), were unsuccessful in alleviating his condition.

Stool specimens were submitted for culture for enteric pathogens and for routine examination for ova and parasites. No enteric bacilli were isolated in culture. No parasites were detected in the routine examination for ova and parasites. The patient's physician then ordered additional tests, including a special stain for coccidia. The laboratory performed a modified acid-fast stain, which revealed small, round, pink structures measuring 4 to 6 μm in diameter (Fig. 6.1).

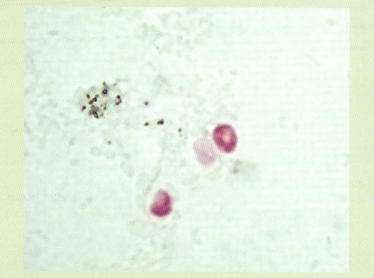

Figure 6.1

QUESTIONS

1. Which protozoan parasite do you suspect of causing this patient's symptoms? Why? What are the "pink structures" seen in the modified acid-fast smear?

2. Explain the classification of this parasite. List related genera that develop in the gastrointestinal tracts of vertebrates throughout their entire life cycles.

3. Describe the life cycle of this parasite.

4. Which other disease-causing coccidian parasites are acid-fast? How might you distinguish them?

5. Are there any other methods available to diagnose this infection?

6. Why will it be difficult to eradicate this parasite from this patient, and why is he at particular risk for developing an intractable infection?

7. How is this infection transmitted?

8. How can this infection be prevented?

ANSWERS

1. The patient is probably infected with *Cryptosporidium parvum*. The modified acid-fast procedure is used to diagnose this infection. The "pink structures" are oocysts of *C. parvum*, which stain pinkish red by this procedure and measure 4 to 6 μm in diameter.

2. *C. parvum* is an intestinal protozoan in the phylum Apicomplexa and is a member of the coccidia. Other coccidian genera which develop in the gastrointestinal tracts of vertebrates throughout their entire life cycles include *Isospora*, *Cyclospora*, and *Eimeria*. These protozoans are nonmotile, obligate intracellular parasites and have complex life cycles. Alternating sexual and asexual stages are usually found in the definitive and the intermediate host, respectively. Coccidia are frequently found in a variety of animals, and certain species are known to infect humans.

3. After ingestion of oocysts of *C. parvum*, sporozoites are released in the upper gastrointestinal tract. The sporozoites are located in the enterocytes of the small intestine and develop further on the brush borders of intestinal epithelial cells. The parasites develop in an intracellular, extracytoplasmic location and are surrounded by host-derived membranes. The parasites are located in vacuoles on the microvillous surface of host cells.

   Asexual reproduction (schizogony) occurs, with the production of merozoites. A cycle of sexual reproduction also occurs, in which microgametes and macrogametes (male and female sex cells, respectively) develop and unite to form zygotes. The zygotes develop into thick-walled oocysts which contain sporozoites. These oocysts, which are infective, pass in the feces and serve as the means of transmission to new hosts. Thin-walled oocysts are also formed and are considered to be responsible for autoinfection. Sporozoites parasitize other intestinal cells and reinitiate the life cycle.

4. *Cyclospora cayetanensis* and *Isospora belli* may resemble *C. parvum*, in that they both stain pink using the modified acid-fast stain. However, the marked difference in size and shape allows them to be differentiated from each other. The oocysts of *Cyclospora* autofluoresce and are slightly larger (8 to 10 μm) than those of *C. parvum*. The modified acid-fast stain usually reveals a variety of oocysts of variable intensity, from colorless to pink to deep red. The oocysts of *I. belli* are much larger (25 to 30 μm) than are those of *C. parvum* and are more ellipsoid. Multiple stool specimens may be needed to make a diagnosis of cryptosporidiosis.

5. Immunoassays including IFA and ELISA are commercially available for the detection of *C. parvum* antigens in the diagnosis of cryptosporidiosis. These methods have excellent sensitivity and result in a higher rate of detection than traditional microscopic assays; they are also less labor-intensive. Immunochromatographic lateral-flow membrane assays, using a cartridge format, are sensitive, specific, rapid, and easy-to-read immunoassays for the diagnosis of cryptosporidiosis. This method relies on capillary action, since parasite antigens are captured by specific antibody as the sample moves laterally through the unit. Combination kits to detect *Giardia lamblia* and *C. parvum* are commercially available.

Although procedures exist for the cultivation of this protozoan parasite in vitro, these methods are labor-intensive, difficult, and expensive and are not useful in the clinical diagnostic laboratory; they are used primarily as research tools rather than diagnostic tools. The Entero-Test capsule may also be used in the diagnosis of cryptosporidiosis (this test is described in case 2). Biopsy specimens taken from the brush border of epithelial cells in the intestine, and sometimes other tissues, may be histologically examined in diagnosing cryptosporidiosis.

6. No good treatment is available for cryptosporidiosis. Recovery from cryptosporidiosis is dependent on a healthy immune system in the host. In patients infected with HIV and in other severely immunocompromised individuals, the infection often becomes progressively worse and frequently does not respond to treatment. The illness may become intractable and may eventually cause death. The presence of thin-walled oocysts, thought to be involved in autoinfection, may explain the overwhelming infections sometimes seen in immunocompromised patients. This patient is particularly at risk, since he is unable to tolerate the "cocktail" of anti-retroviral drugs used to treat HIV infection. It has recently been noted that AIDS patients being treated with these agents to enhance their immune response are less likely to suffer severe, symptomatic, systemic cryptosporidiosis than are severely immunocompromised patients.

Other body sites in addition to the gastrointestinal tract, such as the respiratory tract, may become infected.

7. Cryptosporidiosis is known to be a zoonosis; cattle act as reservoirs of infection. The mature resistant thick-walled oocyst of *C. parvum* is passed in the feces of humans or animals and serves as the infective form for new hosts. Infection usually occurs when food or water contaminated with infective oocysts is ingested. However, person-to-person contact may also transmit disease. Waterborne outbreaks frequently occur. Oocysts are found worldwide and are present in most untreated water supplies. Oocysts of *C. parvum* are difficult to remove physically, requiring filtration, and are resistant to chlorine and many other chemicals.

8. Infection with *C. parvum* can be prevented by adequate disposal of human waste, proper water treatment, and use of good sanitary practices, including improved hygiene and washing of contaminated foods such as fruits and vegetables. It is essential to treat water supplies by filtration techniques in addition to using chemicals. Avoidance of contact with animals, especially by immunocompromised individuals, should reduce the incidence of cryptosporidiosis.

Case 7   A 5-year-old girl had been suffering from intermittent diarrhea, nausea, general malaise, and unexplained loss of appetite and had complained of a stomach ache. The child was in nursery school and had recently been diagnosed with a pinworm infection. She had been treated for this infection and seemed to make a full recovery. Her pediatrician ordered laboratory tests, including a complete blood count, a stool culture, and three stool specimens for examination for ova and parasites.

Slight eosinophilia was reported. The stool culture was negative for enteric bacterial pathogens. The slides of the concentrated specimens for ova and parasites were negative for all three specimens. Two of the three permanent smears stained by the trichrome method were reported negative; the third specimen showed a few protozoan trophozoites (Fig. 7.1). Each trophozoite measured 7 to 14 μm, and appeared slightly rounded. Although two nuclei were present in most trophozoites seen, some of the cells had only a single nucleus. A delicate nuclear membrane was only slightly visible. The nuclear chromatin was fragmented into four or five chromatin granules located symmetrically. Peripheral nuclear chromatin was absent. Vacuoles containing bacteria were present in the cytoplasm.

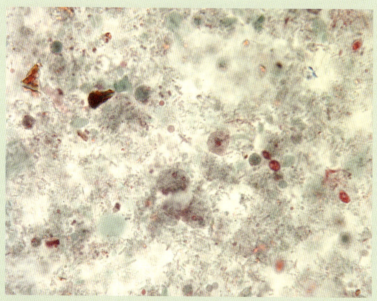

Figure 7.1

QUESTIONS

1. Which intestinal protozoan parasite fits the description given? What is the nature of the confusion surrounding the classification of this parasite?

2. What may be the association of pinworm infection with this patient's present infection?

3. In addition to this parasite, which other parasitic infections are common in nursery schools?

4. Would you expect to find cysts as well as trophozoites in the stool specimen?

5. Why do you think that the protozoa were not visible in any of the sediments prepared from the fecal concentrates but were present in the permanent trichrome smear prepared from only one of the specimens? Why is careful examination of permanent stained smears essential to diagnose this infection?

6. How did the results of blood tests support the diagnosis of this infection?

7. This patient was suffering from a variety of symptoms, including diarrhea. Should you look for this parasite in formed stools?

8. Should this patient be treated? How?

9. Discuss the life cycle of this parasite.

ANSWERS

1. *Dientamoeba fragilis*. The classification of this protozoan is controversial. It was originally classified as an ameba, due to its roundish shape and its propensity to move in ameboid fashion by means of broad, hyaline pseudopods with serrated edges. It is currently classified as a flagellate or as an ameboflagellate due to its structure and progressive style of motility. It is, however, quite difficult to recognize this parasite in a wet-preparation examination of a stool sediment. Although no external flagella are visible, studies utilizing electron microscopic techniques suggest that internal flagella are present.

2. This protozoan is thought to be transmitted in the ova of certain helminths, including *Enterobius vermicularis* (pinworm) and *Ascaris lumbricoides*. This hypothesis, not yet proven, is based on the frequency of finding *D. fragilis* in patients infected with these helminths, as well as the detection by electron microscopy of structures resembling pinworm eggs containing *D. fragilis*.

3. In addition to dientamoebiasis, giardiasis and cryptosporidiosis are common in nursery schools. This is not surprising, since these parasites are usually transmitted by the fecal-oral route.

4. No. *D. fragilis* produces only trophozoites, and no cyst form is known to exist.

5. This parasite can easily be missed, even in the permanent stained smear. The trophozoites are delicate and may be pale-staining and difficult to visualize. There is considerable variation in size and shape of the trophozoites. Several specimens should be tested, since intermittent passage of parasites has been reported. Although procedures exist for the cultivation of this protozoan parasite in vitro, these methods are labor-intensive, difficult, and expensive and are not useful in the clinical diagnostic laboratory; they are used primarily as research tools rather than diagnostic tools. It is necessary to examine the permanent stained smear for pale-staining trophozoites with one or two nuclei (hence the name *Dientamoeba*). Trophozoites having one nucleus may be confused with those of *Entamoeba hartmanni* or *Endolimax nana*. Careful examination of a permanent stained smear is

essential for diagnosis, since the parasite tends to stain weakly, often blending into the background.

6. Although a high eosinophil count usually suggests helminthic infection, peripheral eosinophilia is common in patients with dientamoebiasis. However, the eosinophilia is not as pronounced as in infections with helminths, especially those whose life cycles include an indirect migration phase. This might be associated with the hypothesis that, as mentioned above, *D. fragilis* may be transmitted in the ova of certain helminths, including *Enterobius vermicularis* and *A. lumbricoides*.

7. Since the trophozoites of this parasite have been recovered from formed stools, specimens should be examined by microscopic observation of a sediment prepared from a concentrated specimen and by a permanent stained smear. The specimen should not be rejected if the stool specimen is neither liquid nor soft.

8. Symptomatic patients with *D. fragilis* infections may show improvement following treatment with paromomycin, metronidazole, tetracycline, or iodoquinol. For children, metronidazole is often used.

9. Since the cyst stage of *D. fragilis* has not been confirmed, it is thought that dientamoebiasis is acquired by ingestion of trophozoites of this parasite. Although the complete life cycle of *D. fragilis* is not well understood, we do know that inside the human body this parasite takes up residence in the mucosal crypts in the large intestine. No tissue invasion occurs. Trophozoites are passed in the feces, and the cycle begins again.

Case 8

A 43-year-old man had recently returned from a month-long trip to New Guinea, where he visited his uncle, who was a pig farmer. He had been suffering from abdominal pain and severe, watery, nonbloody diarrhea since returning to the United States from the trip. He visited his family physician in search of a diagnosis.

Since his symptoms were consistent with a diagnosis of dysentery, stool specimens were sent to the laboratory for culture for bacterial pathogens, including *Shigella dysenteriae*, which causes bacillary dysentery, and a routine examination for intestinal parasites, including *Entamoeba histolytica*, which causes amebic dysentery. The culture was negative for enteric bacterial pathogens. The permanent trichrome-stained smear was negative for parasites. However, a moderate number of large bean-shaped ciliated trophozoites were seen microscopically on the wet preparation made from the concentrated stool specimen. A typical parasite is shown in Fig. 8.1.

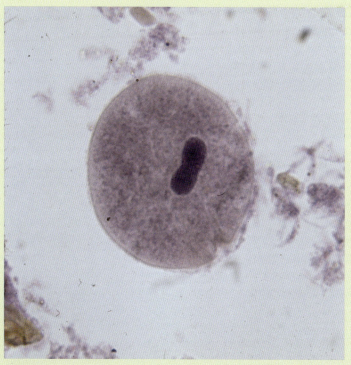

Figure 8.1

QUESTIONS

1. Which protozoan parasite would fit the morphological description of the parasite observed in the microscopic wet mount? What is this condition called?

2. Describe the appearance of characteristic trophozoites of this parasite.

3. Describe the appearance of characteristic cysts of this parasite.

4. Why do you think the permanent trichrome stained smear was negative for this parasite?

5. What might be the relationship between the patient's recent trip to New Guinea and his subsequent infection?

6. How is infection with this parasite transmitted?

7. How would infection with this parasite be prevented?

8. Can this parasite cause the same type of extraintestinal infection associated with *Entamoeba histolytica?* Explain your answer.

9. Which drugs might be effective in treating this patient?

ANSWERS

1. The large, bean-shaped, ciliated structures are trophozoites of the ciliate *Balantidium coli.* The condition is called balantidiasis. Abscesses and ulcers may form in the mucosa and submucosa of the large intestine when infection is severe. This condition may resemble amebic dysentery. This parasite is the only pathogenic intestinal ciliate, and it is the largest intestinal protozoan parasite that causes gastrointestinal disease in humans.

2. The oval trophozoites of *B. coli* are large, measuring 50 to 100 μm in length, and 40 to 70 μm in width. A cytostome is located at the anterior end, which is tapered. Each trophozoite contains two nuclei. One of these is a large, kidney-shaped macronucleus; the other nucleus is a small, round micronucleus, often difficult to see, located next to the macronucleus. Cilia, which are usually longer at the anterior end, are located around the periphery of the trophozoite. Contractile vacuoles are often present in the cytoplasm. The excretory pore, which is called a cytopyge, is located opposite the cytostome. The cytoplasm may contain ingested bacteria.

Although procedures exist for the cultivation of this protozoan parasite in vitro, these methods are labor-intensive, difficult, and expensive and are not useful in the clinical diagnostic laboratory; they are used primarily as research tools rather than diagnostic tools.

3. The cysts of *B. coli* are round to oval and measure 45 to 65 μm. Each cyst contains a large kidney-shaped macronucleus. A small round micronucleus, which is hard to see, is present next to the macronucleus. Cilia, which may be absent in mature cysts, are located within the two layers of the cyst wall.

4. Because of the large size of the trophozoites and cysts of *B. coli,* parasites may be difficult to recognize on a permanent stained smear. Smears are often dark, obscuring the morphology of the parasite. Wet preparations of concentrated stool specimens or fresh material are recommended for detection of this parasite.

5. This patient's uncle was a farmer who had a close association with pigs. Pigs are known to serve as reservoirs for this parasite. Although rarely encountered in the United States, *B. coli* is found in pigs in warm and temperate climates and is known to be endemic in New Guinea.

6. Outbreaks of balantidiasis are rare. Transmission of *B. coli* usually occurs following the ingestion of cysts in food or water which has been contaminated, sometimes by infected food handlers.

7. Balantidiasis may be prevented by improving personal hygiene practices and sanitary methods to reduce fecal-oral transmission. Since pigs are known reservoirs for the parasite, individuals should be aware of the potential risks associated with these animals.

8. Trophozoites of *Entamoeba histolytica* may invade the wall of the colon, enter the circulation, and spread hematogenously to other areas of the body. In addition to causing liver abscesses, *E. histolytica* may affect other areas, including the lungs, spleen, and brain. In rare cases, *B. coli* causes extraintestinal infection, spreading to the lungs, liver, and other organs.

9. The antimicrobial agent tetracycline is considered to be the drug of choice for treatment of infection with *B. coli*. However, its use for this purpose is considered to be investigational. Metronidazole and iodoquinol may also be used.

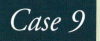

Case 9

A 3-year-old girl was brought to her pediatrician by her mother, who was concerned about the child's diarrhea of 1 week's duration. She had also vomited several times. The girl attended a day care center while her mother was at work. The pediatrician ordered stool specimens for culture for enteric pathogens and for routine examination for ova and parasites.

No enteric pathogens were isolated in culture. Microscopic examination of concentrated sediments of the stool specimens was negative for ova and parasites. No parasites were detected in the permanent trichrome smears. When the results of these tests were received, the pediatrician ordered a special stain for coccidia. The modified acid-fast stain (Fig. 9.1) revealed pinkish red round to oval structures, 4 to 6 μm in diameter.

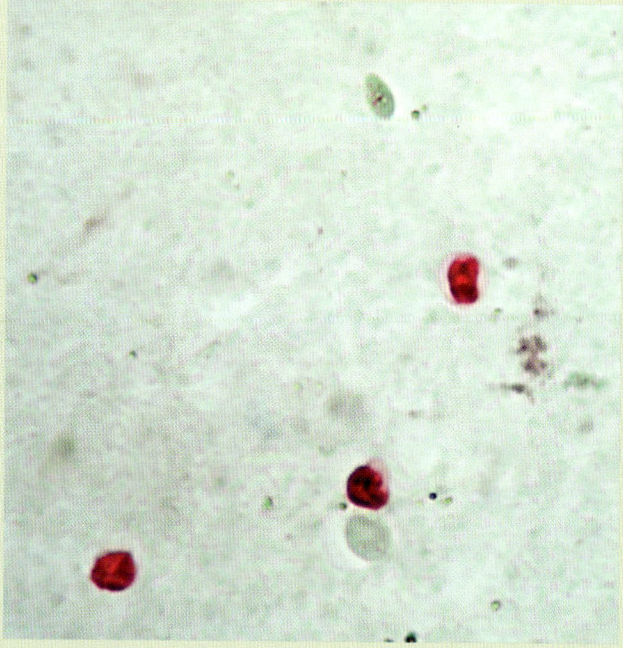

Figure 9.1

QUESTIONS

1. Which protozoan parasite do you think was causing this patient's illness? Explain.

2. Which other procedures may be used to diagnosis this infection?

3. Which factor in the child's history might put her at risk for such infections? Which other parasitic infections are associated with this factor?

4. Why would this patient's course of illness probably be less severe than the same infection in an AIDS patient?

5. Should this child be treated? How?

6. Describe the life cycle of this parasite.

7. There are two other coccidian parasites that are modified acid-fast. Name these parasites, and explain how you would distinguish them from the parasite infecting this child.

ANSWERS

1. The patient is infected with *Cryptosporidium parvum*. The modified acid-fast procedure may be used to diagnose this infection. Oocysts of *C. parvum* stain pinkish red using this procedure and measure 4 to 6 μm in diameter.

2. IFA and ELISA are commercially available immunoassays used for the detection of *Cryptosporidium* antigens in the diagnosis of cryptosporidiosis. These methods have excellent sensitivity and result in a higher rate of detection than traditional microscopic assays; they are also less labor-intensive. Immunochromatographic lateral-flow membrane assays for *C. parvum*, using a cartridge format, are sensitive, specific, rapid, and easy-to-read immunoassays for the diagnosis of cryptosporidiosis. This method relies on capillary action, since parasite antigens are captured by specific antibody as the sample moves laterally through the unit. Combination kits to detect *Giardia lamblia* and *C. parvum* are also commercially available.

   Although procedures exist for the cultivation of this protozoan parasite in vitro, these methods are labor-intensive, difficult, and expensive and are not useful in the clinical diagnostic laboratory; they are used primarily as research tools rather than diagnostic tools. The Entero-Test capsule may also be used in the diagnosis of cryptosporidiosis (this test is described in case 2). Biopsy specimens taken from the brush border of epithelial cells in the intestine, and sometimes other tissues, may be histologically examined in diagnosing cryptosporidiosis.

3. The fact that the child attended a day care center is a risk factor for acquiring cryptosporidiosis, since *C. parvum* causes diarrheal disease in children attending nurseries and day care centers. Person-to-person fecal-oral transmission of infection from young children with cryptosporidiosis frequently occurs. Babies wearing diapers are an especially common source of environmental contamination.

   In addition to cryptosporidiosis, dientamoebiasis and giardiasis are common in nursery schools. This is not surprising since these parasites are usually transmitted by the fecal-oral route. A helminthic infection caused by the nematode *Enterobius vermicularis* (pinworm) is frequently diagnosed in this population, as well.

4. Cryptosporidiosis is usually self-limited in immunocompetent individuals but may be severe in immunocompromised patients such as those with AIDS. Recovery from cryptosporidiosis is dependent on a healthy immune system in the host. In patients infected with HIV and in other severely immunocompromised individuals, the infection often becomes much worse and frequently does not respond to treatment. These patients may develop a secretory diarrhea, associated with massive fluid and electrolyte loss, with subsequent dehydration. The illness may become intractable and eventually may cause death. The presence of thin-walled oocysts, thought to be involved in autoinfection, may explain the overwhelming infections sometimes seen in immunocompromised patients.

5. The illness would probably be self-limited in this otherwise healthy child. Adequate hydration should be maintained as needed. No good treatment is available for cryptosporidiosis.

6. After ingestion of oocysts of *C. parvum*, sporozoites are released in the upper gastrointestinal tract. The sporozoites are located in the enterocytes of the small intestine and develop further on the brush borders of intestinal epithelial cells. The parasites develop in an intracellular, extracytoplasmic location and are surrounded by host-derived membranes. The parasites are located in vacuoles on the microvillous surface of host cells.

Asexual reproduction (schizogony) occurs, with the production of merozoites. A cycle of sexual reproduction also occurs, in which microgametes and macrogametes (male and female sex cells, respectively) develop and unite to form zygotes. The zygotes develop into thick-walled oocysts which contain sporozoites. These oocysts, which are infective, pass in the feces and serve as the means of transmission to new hosts. Thin-walled oocysts are also formed and are considered to be responsible for autoinfection. Sporozoites parasitize other intestinal cells and reinitiate the life cycle.

7. *Cyclospora cayetanensis* and *Isospora belli* may be confused with *Cryptosporidium parvum*, since they all stain pink to red using the modified acid-fast stain. The oocysts of *Cyclospora* autofluoresce and are slightly larger (8 to 10 μm) than those of *C. parvum*. The modified acid-fast stain usually reveals a variety of oocysts, of variable intensity, from colorless to pink to deep red. The oocysts of *Isospora belli* are much larger (25 to 30 μm) than the oocysts of *C. parvum* and are more ellipsoid. Multiple stool specimens may be needed to make a diagnosis.

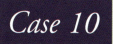

A 45-year-old man had been suffering from diarrhea, nausea, vomiting, and abdominal discomfort for 1 month before visiting his primary-care physician. Stool specimens were collected and submitted for routine bacterial culture and examination for ova and parasites. No enteric bacterial pathogens grew in culture. A saline wet mount prepared by concentration techniques revealed rare "central-body" parasitic forms which measured 7 to 12 μm. These refractile structures contained large, clear, central areas resembling vacuoles, surrounded by several granules around the periphery. A permanent smear stained by the trichrome method showed a moderate number of intensely stained blue, vacuolated central-body forms (Fig. 10.1), measuring 8 to 12 μm, with purplish peripheral granules. In addition, a few amebic trophozoites, measuring 8 to 10 μm, with evenly distributed peripheral nuclear chromatin, were seen.

The report from the parasitology laboratory read, "Ova and Parasitology examination revealed *Entamoeba hartmanni* and moderate *Blastocystis hominis*."

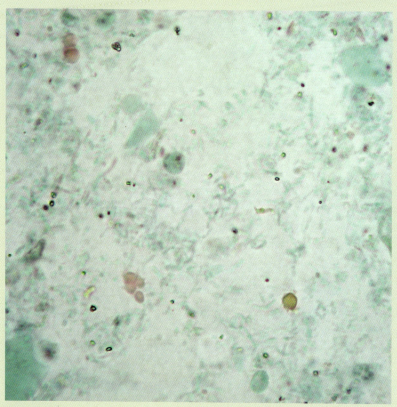

Figure 10.1

QUESTIONS

1. Could either of the parasites listed above be the cause of this patient's diarrhea? Explain.

2. What explanation can you give for the difference in quantity of *Blastocystis hominis* seen in the saline wet mount and in the permanent trichrome stain?

3. What accounts for the uncertain taxonomic situation of *Blastocystis hominis?*

4. Describe the life cycle of *Blastocystis hominis.*

5. Which treatment might be given for this infection? How would the treatment differ from that of *Entamoeba histolytica?*

6. Discuss the epidemiology and prevention of this infection.

ANSWERS

1. *Entamoeba hartmanni* is nonpathogenic and would not be causing this patient's symptoms. Although *Blastocystis hominis* is commonly found as a normal resident of the intestinal tract in healthy asymptomatic carriers, it may cause gastrointestinal symptoms when present in moderate to large numbers in symptomatic patients. It has been suggested that different strains of *B. hominis* exist. Some strains may be pathogenic; others may be nonpathogenic. This may explain why some patients infected with this parasite are asymptomatic.

When *B. hominis* is identified, the specimen should be carefully examined for other pathogenic parasites. When such microorganisms are detected, these agents should be considered to be the most likely cause of the patient's symptoms. At least three specimens for ova and parasites should be collected to rule out any other pathogenic protozoa before concluding that a patient's symptoms are caused by *B. hominis*.

2. It is known that *B. hominis* organisms may be ruptured by contact with water. Therefore, rinsing of the stool specimen, as suggested for certain concentration procedures, is not recommended for any of the protozoa, but especially for detection of this parasite. Saline may sometimes lyse the cells, which may explain the rarity of the parasite in the saline wet mount prepared from the stool specimen from this patient. Stool specimens should be placed in a preservative before the concentration procedure is performed. As with all protozoan parasites, microscopic examination should include a permanent stain, such as the trichrome or iron hematoxylin stain, which is the method of choice to detect infection with *B. hominis*.

Although procedures exist for the cultivation of this protozoan parasite in vitro, these methods are labor-intensive, difficult, and expensive and are not useful in the clinical diagnostic laboratory; they are used primarily as research tools rather than diagnostic tools.

3. *B. hominis* is of uncertain taxonomic affiliation, probably because of the different morphologic forms of this parasite that are known to exist. In addition to the vacuolated, central-body form seen in this patient, a more amebic form may also be seen. It is easily confused with other protozoa and with yeast cells. Although this parasite is able to form pseudopods, it reproduces by binary fission or sporulation. At various times classified as a yeast, as a cyst form of a flagellate, and as a protozoan sporozoan, it has recently been classified as a stramenopile. Suggestions have been made to create a new class and a new order for this microorganism. Ongoing molecular studies may result in its reclassification in the future.

4. The life cycle of *B. hominis* has not been fully described. However, stages of this parasite appear to include the amebic form, the cyst form, and the vacuolated central-body form. The central-body form is the one usually found in human feces, although diarrheal stool specimens occasionally reveal the amebic form. Although the parasite reproduces by binary fission or sporulation, the central body is also involved in sexual and asexual reproduction. Bacteria and debris in the intestine serve as nutrients for *B. hominis*.

5. Metronidazole may be used to treat *B. hominis* in symptomatic patients when the parasite is present in moderate to large numbers. Iodoquinol is an alternate choice. These antimicrobial agents may also be used to treat infections with *Entamoeba histolytica*. However, a patient with even a small number of *E. histolytica* organisms should be treated to avoid the spread of this parasite to noninfected individuals.

6. Infection with *B. hominis* occurs worldwide, and the parasite is transmitted by the fecal-oral route. Contaminated food or water appears to be the vehicle of infection. This infection could be prevented by improved personal hygiene, the washing of contaminated fruits and vegetables before eating, and the adequate disposal of human waste.

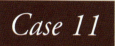

Case 11

A 32-year-old woman with pain in her right eye was seen by her ophthalmologist, who diagnosed a corneal ulcer in the affected eye. Her physical examination was unremarkable otherwise; she had no history of eye problems and had recently been examined by her primary-care physician, who declared her to be in good health.

Bacterial cultures taken from a discharge from her eye were negative. Viral cultures were also negative. Specimens were collected for culture for free-living amebae. No amebic parasite was recovered in culture. Figure 11.1 shows the parasite in a smear stained by the chromotrope Gram stain method. The Warthin-Starry silver stain was used to confirm the diagnosis.

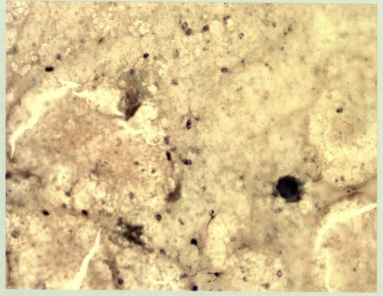

Figure 11.1

QUESTIONS

1. Which group of obligate intracellular protozoan parasites fits the description given and might be causing this infection in this immunocompetent woman?

2. List several members of this group that may be causing this patient's infection.

3. Which laboratory procedure may be used to identify the parasite to genus level?

4. What are the structures seen in the smear?

5. Which other laboratory procedures are available to diagnose infections with this group of protozoans?

6. Describe the pathogenesis of this infection.

7. How does this infection differ in immunocompromised (AIDS) patients?

ANSWERS

1. The obligate intracellular protozoan parasite was probably a member of the phylum Microspora. These parasites, long known to be parasites in invertebrates, have increasingly been recognized as opportunistic pathogens in patients with AIDS. However, they also have also been found in patients with healthy immune systems.

2. Several microsporidian parasites, including *Vittaforma corneae, Nosema ocularum,* and *Microsporidium* species, have been associated with keratitis or corneal ulcers in immunocompetent patients. These infections are sometimes associated with some form of prior trauma to the eye.

3. Electron microscopy may be used to help in the identification of the microsporidia to genus level. Although this procedure is highly specific, it is labor-intensive and lacks the sensitivity of other methods.

4. The structures seen in the smear are environmentally resistant microsporidian spores, which measure 1 to 5 μm, about the size of a bacterial cell. Each spore contains a coiled, tubular extrusion apparatus (polar tubule or filament). The polar tubule is extruded forcefully when contact is made with adjacent host cells. It penetrates a host cell, and the contents of the spore (sporoplasm) are then injected into the cytoplasm of the host cell.

5. Microsporidiosis may be diagnosed by the identification of spores in biopsy material, by the Giemsa stain, and by the histological periodic acid-Schiff stain. Specimens may also be stained by the chromotrope Gram stain or the modified trichrome stain. Several formulations of this stain, including the Weber green and the Ryan blue modified trichrome stains, are commercially available. Since penetration of the stain into the spore wall is difficult, the staining time is much longer than in the traditional trichrome stain method. However, heating the stain to 50°C decreases the staining time and greatly increases the quality of the stain.

Chemofluorescent (optical brightening) agents are useful in the detection of *Enterocytozoon bieneusi* spores. Using Calcofluor White, the spores may be seen under a fluorescence microscope. These agents, although sensitive for the detection of microsporidia, are not specific for these organisms. Routine hematoxylin and eosin stains are difficult to read.

Although procedures exist for the cultivation of these protozoan parasites in vitro, these methods are labor-intensive, difficult, and expensive and are not useful in the clinical diagnostic laboratory. These methods are used primarily as research tools rather than diagnostic tools.

6. Ocular infection in the immunocompetent host is classified pathologically as stromal keratitis and usually leads to corneal ulcers. The microsporidia are located deep in the corneal stroma. Spores of the organisms are usually both free and contained within phagocytic cells. Inflammation is intense and is characterized by neutrophilic, mononuclear, and epithelioid infiltrates.

7. In immunocompromised (AIDS) patients, ocular infection is classified as epithelial, since the microsporidia (usually *Encephalitozoon* species) are found in the superficial epithelial cells of the cornea or conjunctiva. Inflammation is mild or absent and is characterized by neutrophilic and mononuclear infiltrates. Microsporidia particularly associated with these patients include *Encephalitozoon cuniculi*, *Encephalitozoon hellem*, and *Encephalitozoon intestinalis*.

<table>
<tr><td>**Case 12**</td><td>A 28-year-old man, who had AIDS and who had had a low CD4 count (50 cells/mm^3) for approximately 1 year, presented to his primary-care physician suffering from diarrhea</td></tr>
</table>

for 10 weeks and a recent weight loss of 20 lb. His diarrhea was watery and profuse but nonbloody. Nonprescription antidiarrheal medications (e.g., loperamide HCl [Imodium]) were not successful in alleviating his condition. The patient showed signs of dehydration on examination. A stool specimen was submitted to the laboratory for routine culture for bacterial pathogens, and three stool specimens, collected on alternate days, were examined for ova and parasites. The routine culture was negative for bacterial pathogens.

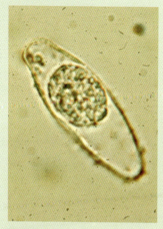

Pale oval structures were seen in the wet preparation from the concentrated sediment (Fig. 12.1). When the permanent stained trichrome smear showed evidence of a protozoan parasite, a special stain for coccidia was performed. A modified acid-fast procedure revealed elliptical pink structures measuring 25 to 30 μm. Each structure was surrounded by a clear, double-layer wall.

Figure 12.1

QUESTIONS

1. Which protozoan parasite do you think is causing this patient's illness? What are the structures seen in the patient's stool specimen?

2. Why was the modified acid-fast procedure needed to definitively identify the parasite?

3. Which other two coccidian parasites give a similar reaction when stained by the modified acid-fast procedure?

4. How would you distinguish these three parasites?

5. Describe the life cycle of the parasite causing this patient's infection.

6. Why would this patient pose less risk to laboratory personnel than patients infected with other coccidian parasites?

7. How is infection with this parasite transmitted?

8. How should this patient be treated?

ANSWERS

1. The protozoan parasite seen in this patient's stool specimen is *Isospora belli*. The elliptical pink structures seen in the modified acid-fast smear are oocysts of this parasite.

2. The oocysts of *I. belli* are often very pale and transparent in the wet mount prepared from the concentrated stool sediment. They may be missed in the permanent stained smear, since they often stain dark and can resemble debris. Wet preparations of concentrated stool specimens or fresh material are recommended for detection of this parasite. The modified acid-fast procedure may also be used.

3. *Cryptosporidium parvum* and *Cyclospora cayetanensis* give similar reactions when stained by the modified acid-fast method. Although all three of the parasites stain pink using the modified acid-fast stain, they may be distinguished by their different shapes and sizes.

4. The oocysts of *Cryptosporidium parvum* measure 4 to 6 μm, while those of *Cyclospora cayetanensis* are about twice as large, measuring 8 to 10 μm. The oocysts of *I. belli* are much larger (25 to 30 μm) than the oocysts of *Cryptosporidium parvum* and *Cyclospora cayetanensis* and are more oval or ellipsoid. The modified acid-fast stain of *Cyclospora cayetanensis* demonstrates oocysts ranging in intensity from unstained, glassy, wrinkled spheres, to light pink or dark red structures. UV techniques used to detect autofluorescence show a weak green or blue fluorescence when *Cyclospora cayetanensis* is present.

5. The life cycle of *I. belli* is similar to that of other coccidia. Stages include the formation of schizonts, merozoites, gametocytes, gametes, and oocysts. The mature, infective oocysts are usually ingested in food or water. Sporozoites are released, and development occurs within the epithelial cells of the small intestine. Asexual reproduction, known as schizogony, results in the formation of merozoites. Macro- and microgametes are formed during the sexual stage of development. The gametes unite to form the immature oocysts, which are passed in the feces. After passage from the host in the feces, the immature oocyst develops into the mature, sporulated oocyst, which is infective for humans.

6. This patient would pose little risk for the development of laboratory-acquired infection, since the oocysts, unlike those of *Cryptosporidium parvum*, are not initially infective. When passed in human feces, the immature oocyst is noninfective and contains a single central mass. After further maturation, the oocyst develops two sporoblasts. These develop into two sporocysts, each of which contains four cigar-shaped sporozoites. A clear, double-layer wall surrounds the mature cyst, which is the infective form.

7. Transmission of *I. belli* occurs by ingestion of water or food containing infective oocysts of the parasite. No zoonotic transmission is known to occur. Cases of isosporiasis have occurred worldwide; however, infection is usually asymptomatic and self-limited. Symptoms of this infection may include diarrhea, abdominal pain, weight loss and anorexia.

Cases of infection in HIV-infected patients have increased in recent years. Extraintestinal infections have occurred in some of these patients. In chronic infections, oocysts may be shed for months or years. Isosporiasis may be prevented by improving personal hygiene practices and sanitary methods to reduce the fecal-oral transmission of this parasite.

8. Individuals without symptoms or with minimal symptoms may not require treatment. The treatment of choice for serious infection with *I. belli* is trimethoprim-sulfamethoxazole.

REFERENCES

Arrowood, M. J. 2002. In vitro cultivation of *Cryptosporidium* species. *Clin. Microbiol. Rev.* **15**:390–400.

Ash, L. R., and T. C. Orihel. 1991. *Parasites: a Guide to Laboratory Procedures and Identification.* ASCP Press, Chicago, Ill.

Blessmann, J., H. Buss, P. A. Nu, B. T. Dinh, Q. T. Ngo, A. L. Van, M. D. Alla, T. F. Jackson, J. I. Ravdin, and E. Tannich. 2002. Real-time PCR for detection and differentiation of *Entamoeba histolytica* and *Entamoeba dispar* in fecal samples. *J. Clin. Microbiol.* **40**:4413–4417.

Bryan, R. T., A. Cali, R. L. Owen, and H. C. Spencer. 1991. Microsporidia: opportunistic pathogens in patients with AIDS, p. 1–26. *In* Y. Sun (ed.), *Progress in Clinical Parasitology,* vol. 2. Field and Wood, Philadelphia, Pa.

Chioralia, G., T. Trammer, H. Kampin, and H. M. Seitz. 1998. Relevant criteria for detecting microsporidia in stool specimens. *J. Clin. Microbiol.* **36**:2279–2283.

Clark, C. G., and L. S. Diamond. 2002. Methods for cultivation of luminal parasitic protists of clinical importance. *Clin. Microbiol. Rev.* **15**:329–341.

Garcia, L. S. 2002. Laboratory identification of the microsporidia. *J. Clin. Microbiol.* **40**:1892–1901.

Garcia, L. S. 2001. *Diagnostic Medical Parasitology,* 4th ed. ASM Press, Washington, D.C.

Heelan, J. S., and F. W. Ingersoll. 2002. *Essentials of Human Parasitology.* Thomson Delmar Learning, Albany, N.Y.

Kokoskin, E., T. W. Gyorkos, A. Camus, L. Cedilotte, T. Purtill, and B. Ward. 1994. Modified technique for efficient detection of microsporidia. *J. Clin. Microbiol.* **32**:1074–1075.

Koneman, E. W., S. D. Allen, W. M. Janda, P. C. Schreckenberger, and W. C. Winn, Jr. 1997. *Color Atlas and Textbook of Diagnostic Microbiology,* 5th ed. Lippincott Publishing, Philadelphia, Pa.

Leber, A. L., and S. M. Novak. 2003. Intestinal and urogenital amebae, flagellates, and ciliates, p. 1990–2007. *In* P. R. Murray, E. J. Baron, J. H. Jorgensen, M. A. Pfaller, and R. H. Yolken (ed.), *Manual of Clinical Microbiology,* 8th ed., vol. 2. ASM Press, Washington, D.C.

Markell, E. K., D. T. John, and W. A. Krotoski. 1999. *Markell and Voge's Medical Parasitology,* 8th ed. The W. B. Saunders Co., Philadelphia, Pa.

Mirelman, D. 1987. Effect of culture conditions and bacterial associates on the zymodemes of *Entamoeba histolytica. Parasitol. Today* **3**:37–40.

Ryan, N. J., G. Sutherland, K. Coughlan, M. Globan, J. Doultree, J. Marshall, R. W. Baird, J. Pedersen, and B. Dwyer. 1993. A new trichrome-blue stain for detection of microsporidial species in urine, stool, and nasopharyngeal specimens. *J. Clin. Microbiol.* **31**:3264–3269.

Shimeld, L., and A. T. Rodgers. 1999. Intestinal and atrial protozoans, p. 572–589. *In* L. Shimeld (ed.), *Essentials of Diagnostic Microbiology.* Thomson Delmar Learning, Albany, N.Y.

Sifuentes-Osornio, J., G. Porras-Cortes, R. P. Bendall, F. Morales-Villarreal, G. Reyes-Teran, and G. M. Ruiz-Palacios. 1995. *Cyclospora cayetanensis* infection in patients with and without AIDS: biliary disease as another clinical manifestation. *Clin. Infect. Dis.* **21**:1092–1097.

Visvesvara, G. S. 2002. In vitro cultivation of microsporidia of clinical importance. *Clin. Microbiol. Rev.* **15**:401–413.

Wolk, D. M., S. K. Schneider, N. L. Wengenack, L. M. Sloan, and J. E. Rosenblatt. 2002. Real-time PCR for detection of *Enterocytozoon intestinalis* from stool specimens. *J. Clin. Microbiol.* **40**:3922–3928.

Wurtz, R. 1994. *Cyclospora*: a newly identified intestinal pathogen of humans. *Clin. Infect. Dis.* **18:**620–623.

Zaki, M., P. Meelu, W. Sun, and C. G. Clark. 2002. Simultaneous differentiation and typing of *Entamoeba histolytica* and *Entamoeba dispar. J. Clin. Microbiol.* **40:**1271–1276.

Zeibig, E. A. 1997. *Clinical Parasitology.* The W. B. Saunders Co., Philadelphia, Pa.

Zierdt, C. H. 1991. *Blastocystis hominis*—past and future. *Clin. Microbiol. Rev.* **4:**61–79.

Zierdt, C. H. 1978. *Blastocystis hominis,* an intestinal protozoan parasite of man. *Public Health Lab.* **36:**147–161.

This section deals with infections caused by blood and tissue protozoa. The free-living amebae, which have been associated with serious infections, are members of this group. This diverse group of protozoans is widespread in the environment, particularly in fresh and salt water, as well as in decaying organic material. Only two genera of these amebae have been implicated in human infection. *Naegleria fowleri* causes a fulminant and rapidly fatal infection of the central nervous system, called primary amebic meningoencephalitis. *Acanthamoeba* species cause amebic keratitis (a chronic infection of the cornea), skin infections, and a more chronic infection of the central nervous system, called granulomatous amebic encephalitis. *Balamuthia mandrillaris* is a recently recognized free-living ameba that also causes granulomatous amebic encephalitis but acts as an opportunist to cause illness, usually in immunocompromised individuals.

Infections caused by the blood and tissue flagellates *Leishmania* species and *Trypanosoma* species are also presented in this section. Unlike intestinal flagellates, hemoflagellates in the genera *Leishmania* and *Trypanosoma* have complex life cycles and are transmitted by blood-sucking invertebrates. Both genera are in the family Trypanosomatidae and are transmitted by insect vectors. Infections caused by *Leishmania* species include cutaneous, mucocutaneous, and visceral leishmaniasis. Cutaneous leishmaniasis causes infections confined to the skin; mucocutaneous leishmaniasis involves mucous membranes, especially the mucous membranes lining the nose and mouth, as well as the skin; and the visceral form of this disease is a systemic infection which may result in the enlargement of internal organs, including the liver and spleen. *Leishmania* species are intracellular parasites of the reticuloendothelial system that are transmitted by phlebotomine sand flies.

The trypanosomes infecting humans include *Trypanosoma brucei* variants *gambiense* and *rhodesiense*, which cause African sleeping sickness, and *Trypanosoma cruzi*, which causes Chagas' disease. *T. brucei gambiense* causes West African trypanosomiasis, and *T. brucei rhodesiense* causes East African trypanosomiasis. The tsetse fly is the vector for African sleeping sickness, while the reduviid bug is the vector for Chagas' disease.

Blood and tissue sporozoa are also included in this section. They include the members of the genus *Plasmodium*, which cause malaria, as well as those causing babesiosis and toxoplasmosis. Malaria is the world's most significant tropical parasitic disease and is responsible for considerable morbidity and mortality worldwide. Protozoans causing malaria are obligate intracellular parasites, with complex life cycles involving sexual and asexual phases, and are transmitted by blood-sucking insect vectors, usually female *Anopheles* mosquitoes.

Babesia species, especially *Babesia microti* in North America, are also obligate intracellular blood parasites that are transmitted by *Ixodes* tick vectors. These deer ticks are also responsible for transmitting Lyme disease and ehrlichiosis. The protozoan that causes babesiosis must be distinguished from the malaria parasite. The ringlike structures characteristic of *B. microti* closely resemble the early stages of the malaria protozoans, especially *Plasmodium falciparum*. Travel history and place of residence are particularly important in making the correct diagnosis in these cases.

Toxoplasmosis is caused by the protozoan *Toxoplasma gondii*. Although most cases of toxoplasmosis are asymptomatic, this parasite poses a great risk to immunocompromised individuals, especially those with AIDS, who may develop cerebral toxoplasmosis, with neurological symptoms. The parasite is also a risk to pregnant women and their developing fetuses. Cats, particularly outdoor cats, are the principal reservoir for *T. gondii*.

Most of the cases presented in this section may be diagnosed by the preparation and examination of thin and thick peripheral blood films. The thick smear may be used as a screen and is especially useful in light infections, while the thin smear is preferred to more clearly visualize morphology and to definitively identify the parasite to species level.

The thin smear is prepared by the push slide technique used to prepare routine blood smears for differential counts in hematology. Using this method, a drop of blood is placed on one end of a glass slide. A second slide, held at a 30° angle, is used to "push" the drop of blood along the slide. The finished smear then has a thick end and a thin, feathered end.

The thick smear is made by placing 2 or 3 drops of blood close together on one end of a glass slide. A corner of another glass slide is used to mix the drops of blood over an area of about 2 cm. The slides must dry completely at room temperature. Thin and thick smears may be stained by the Giemsa or Wright method.

Therapy for infections caused by blood and tissue protozoa varies and may require prolonged treatment with toxic drugs. A wide variety of drugs are available, and the choice may depend on the stage of illness. Treatment of malaria may be particularly complex, especially since *P. falciparum* has developed resistance to some agents. Several blood and tissue parasites do not respond to therapy; the outcome in these situations is grave.

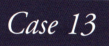

Case 13

A previously healthy 10-year-old boy was seen in July in the emergency department suffering from fever and a severe headache of several days' duration. He had vomited several times and complained of nausea and a runny nose. The weather had been very hot, and the child had spent much of the summer swimming in a local pond. On examination, the emergency room physician noted neck stiffness and performed a lumbar puncture. Cerebrospinal fluid (CSF) was collected and sent to the laboratory for cell count, glucose and protein levels, bacterial culture, and a request to "rule out an amebic infection."

The white blood cell count of the CSF was 25,000 per mm³, with neutrophils predominating. A small number of red blood cells were also present. The glucose level was decreased (<5 mg/dl), and the protein level was markedly elevated (600 mg/dl). The Gram stain of the CSF showed many white blood cells but no bacteria. A wet mount microscopic examination revealed motile amebic trophozoites. A trichrome stain was made and revealed an ameboid form.

A diagnosis of meningoencephalitis was made. The child was admitted to the pediatric intensive care unit but died on the fourth day of hospitalization.

QUESTIONS

1. Which ameba is likely to be responsible for the child's symptoms? What is the name of this infection?

2. What is the correlation between a "hot summer" and the child's illness?

3. What are the stages in the life cycle of this parasite?

4. How is the diagnosis of this infection made in the laboratory?

5. How is this infection transmitted?

6. Which other ameba resembles this parasite and may cause a similar type of infection?

7. How can these two amebae be distinguished?

8. Which other infectious disease might be confused with this illness?

9. Is this infection treatable?

ANSWERS

1. *Naegleria fowleri* is the free-living thermophilic ameboflagellate which is causing this child's infection. The infection, which is rare and usually results in a fulminant and rapidly fatal illness, is called primary amebic meningoencephalitis (PAM).

2. Trophozoites of *N. fowleri* may be found in freshwater sources, including lakes, ponds, streams, hot springs, irrigation ditches, and swimming pools. Although infection is usually associated with swimming, one reported case has involved an infant who had been bathed with well water from which trophozoites of the parasite had been isolated.

The "hot summer" would be responsible for keeping the temperature of local water sources, such as ponds and lakes, very high. When the temperature of these water sources is elevated, this condition leads to increased levels of bacteria. It is known that the concentrations of *N. fowleri* are higher under these conditions, since these amebae feed on the bacteria present. PAM, although rare, causes a rapidly progressive, fatal illness in healthy children and young adults, who have a history of swimming or diving in local water sources in warm weather. The fact that the boy spent much of the summer "swimming in the local pond" supports the diagnosis of meningoencephalitis caused by *N. fowleri*.

3. There are three stages in the life cycle of *N. fowleri,* including both ameboid and flagellate stages. These stages include an amebic trophozoite, a flagellated form possessing two flagella, and a resistant cyst stage. The cyst stage, found in the environment, is not seen in humans.

4. Although trophozoites may be seen in a counting chamber, they are easily missed. A wet mount on a regular slide, with a coverslip, is the recommended method used to make a diagnosis. Examination of a wet mount prepared from fresh CSF usually reveals the characteristic motile ameboid trophozoites of *N. fowleri*. To enhance contrast, it is important to reduce the light. A trichrome-stained smear may also be examined for parasites. The trophozoite has a "sluglike" shape, having a broad anterior end and a narrow posterior end. It measures 7 to 20 μm and has large, broad pseudopods and a single nucleus. The large, central karyosome is not usually visible. No peripheral nuclear chromatin is present. The CSF should not be refrigerated, since the amebae are more actively motile at room temperature. Care must be taken to distinguish these trophozoites from leukocytes.

The amebae may be cultured by seeding agar plates with bacterial cells of *Escherichia coli,* which serve as nutrients, before inoculating the media with the patient's CSF. The agar plates are incubated at 37°C and examined daily for the telltale tracks which are seen in areas of bacterial growth

An indirect immunofluorescence assay may be used to confirm the diagnosis. PCR techniques are not routinely performed in most clinical laboratories but are available at the Centers for Disease Control and Prevention (CDC) laboratories. Consult with your state or county public health laboratory for guidance in submitting specimens to CDC.

5. Transmission of *N. fowleri* occurs when the amebae enter the nose and penetrate the mucous membranes and paranasal sinuses, causing rhinorrhea. The force of water entering the nares when diving into water enables the amebae to pass through lesions or abrasions of the mucous membranes of the nares and enter the tissue. The trophozoites pass through the cribriform plate of the ethmoid bone and follow the olfactory nerve to the central nervous system (CNS). Multiplication of the amebae occurs in tissues of the brain and meninges.

6. Trophozoites of *Acanthamoeba* species resemble those of *Naegleria fowleri* and may cause a chronic CNS infection called granulomatous amebic encephalitis (GAE). Although this infection may lead to death, it does not progress as quickly as fulminant infections caused by *N. fowleri*. *Acanthamoeba* species may also cause an eye infection known as *Acanthamoeba* keratitis, which is not fatal.

7. In *Acanthamoeba* infections, both trophozoites and cysts are found in tissues, while in infections with *N. fowleri*, only trophozoites are found. Trophozoites of *Acanthamoeba* species characteristically have spiky projections (acanthopodia) on their pseudopods, unlike the blunt pseudopods of *N. fowleri*.

8. This disease may be confused with aseptic meningitis or bacterial meningitis, illnesses that have symptoms similar to PAM but are caused by a number of bacterial species. When a large number of white blood cells but no bacteria are seen on Gram stain, a diagnosis of *N. fowleri* infection should be considered.

9. Antimicrobial therapy is usually ineffective against *N. fowleri*. Although *N. fowleri* is very susceptible to amphotericin B in vitro, very few patients recover from this infection. Patients have been successfully treated with intrathecal and intravenous injections of amphotericin B alone, in combination with miconazole, with rifampin and chloramphenicol, or with oral rifampin and ketoconazole.

Case 14

A 24-year-old male medical student from West Africa had lived in the United States for several years and had made periodic visits home to visit his family. When he fell ill with symptoms of severe myalgia, abdominal discomfort, vomiting, diarrhea, fever, chills, and sweats, he presented to the emergency room, where he was noted to have an itchy rash and a tender, indurated, erythematous lesion on his left forearm. He had a diminished reaction to pain. Enlarged posterior cervical lymph nodes were apparent on physical examination.

Blood was drawn for laboratory studies. Based on clinical symptoms and the patient's former residence in West Africa, the laboratory was asked to look for blood parasites. Thick and thin blood smears were prepared and stained by the Giemsa method. A lymph node aspirate was also stained by the Giemsa method. Slender protozoan forms having long, free flagella, were seen in both blood smears and lymph node preparations. Characteristic parasites are shown in Fig. 14.1.

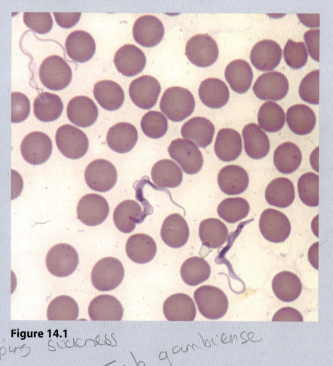

Figure 14.1

QUESTIONS

1. Which infection does this patient have? What is the name of the hemoflagellate causing his infection?

2. Describe the life cycle of this hemoflagellate.

3. What is the term given to the lymphadenopathy noted in this patient?

4. What is the term used to describe the delayed sensation to pain?

5. How is the diagnosis of this infection made?

6. Which form of this parasite is the diagnostic stage seen in clinical specimens? Describe the morphological appearance of this form.

7. How does the patient's travel history aid in the diagnosis of this infection?

8. Discuss the treatment for this infection.

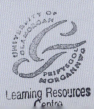

Learning Resources Centre

ANSWERS

1. The patient has West African trypanosomiasis (African sleeping sickness) caused by the hemoflagellate *Trypanosoma brucei gambiense.*

2. Infection with *T. brucei gambiense,* an extracellular parasite, is transmitted when an infected tsetse fly injects saliva containing metacyclic trypomastigotes into the bloodstream of a human host. The hemoflagellates multiply in the tissues surrounding the bite site, pass into the lymphatic system, and then enter the bloodstream. The parasites transform into bloodstream trypomastigotes and are carried to sites throughout the body. Eventually the trypomastigotes reach the CNS, proliferate, and lead to symptoms of disease. Replication occurs by binary fission. The tsetse fly becomes infected while feeding on an infected mammalian host. In the midgut of the fly, the parasites transform into long, slender procyclic trypomastigotes, multiply by binary fission, and develop into epimastigotes in the salivary glands of the tsetse fly, continuing to multiply. Infective metacyclic forms develop in the salivary glands. The life cycle in the tsetse fly lasts about 3 weeks. The tsetse fly remains infective for life.

Although the typical mode of transmission is through the bite of an infected tsetse fly, as described above, rare cases of infections transmitted during blood transfusions or acquired congenitally have been reported.

3. Although any lymph node may be infected by trypanosomes, cervical lymph node involvement is most common. The enlargement of lymph nodes in the posterior cervical region is known as Winterbottom's sign.

4. Severe pain may be experienced a short time after the release of pressure on the palms of the hands or on the ulnar nerve. Kerandel's sign is the term used to describe the delayed sensation to pain.

5. Diagnosis of infection with *T. brucei gambiense* is more difficult than infection with *T. brucei rhodesiense* due to low levels of trypanosomes often associated with the former parasite. Also, numbers of circulating parasites vary and are greater during febrile periods. It is important to take multiple blood specimens to increase the likelihood of making a diagnosis.

Trypanosomes of *T. brucei gambiense* may be demonstrated in thick or thin blood smears stained by the Giemsa method. Concentration of the specimen may be useful if no parasites are seen in these smears. A centrifuged specimen of cerebrospinal fluid or buffy coat may also be examined for characteristic trypanomastigotes. Parasites may also be detected in aspirates of lymph nodes and the trypanosomal chancres.

Serological methods are available but are of limited use in making a diagnosis of West African trypanosomiasis.

6. The trypomastigote is the diagnostic stage seen in clinical specimens, including blood, lymph node aspirates, and CSF. When stained with Giemsa or Wright stain, smears reveal parasites with pale blue cytoplasm and dark blue granules. The nucleus is centrally located and stains reddish. The reddish kinetoplast is located posteriorly. The kinetoplast is smaller than that seen in *T. cruzi*, the causative agent of Chagas' disease, which helps to distinguish the two protozoans. The geographical distribution of these parasites also precludes confusion between them.

A flagellum and an undulating membrane arise from the kinetoplast. The flagellum runs anteriorly and forms the edge of the undulating membrane and then extends anteriorly beyond the body. Unlike *T. cruzi*, which may be present intracellularly as amastigotes or extracellularly as trypomastigotes, *T. brucei gambiense* is present only extracellularly in the trypomastigote form.

7. The patient had made periodic visits to West Africa. The trypomastigotes of *T. brucei gambiense* and *T. brucei rhodesiense* are morphologically identical. However, *T. brucei gambiense* is found in large areas of West and Central Africa and causes West African trypanosomiasis, while *T. brucei rhodesiense* is found in East and Southeast Africa and causes East African trypanosomiasis. It is therefore important to elicit the patient's travel history to make a correct diagnosis.

8. Treatment of African trypanosomiasis requires prolonged administration of toxic drugs. Pentamidine, which does not pass the blood-brain barrier, may be used to treat infections not involving the CNS. Other agents which are effective in treating the hemolymphatic stage and CNS disease caused by *T. brucei gambiense* include suramin and melarsoprol, which is recommended for late-stage disease. Eflornithine may be used to treat melarsoprol-resistant *T. brucei gambiense* infection with or without neural involvement. Patients who do not respond to melarsoprol may be treated with nifurtimox either alone, which may result in relapse, or in combination with melarsoprol.

A 24-year-old male Pakistani medical resident was seen in the emergency department at midnight; he was acutely ill with weakness, fever, abdominal pain, and diarrhea. He had visited relatives in Pakistan several months earlier. He had recently lost 20 lb inexplicably. Physical examination revealed hepatomegaly, splenomegaly, and lymphadenopathy. The patient had darkened areas of skin on his forehead and around his mouth.

Based on the patient's symptoms and travel history, blood tests were ordered to rule out infection with a hemoflagellate. Laboratory tests, including routine hematology tests, revealed that the patient was anemic, with a hemoglobin level of 10 g/dl. He also suffered from leukopenia and thrombocytopenia. Liver enzyme levels were slightly elevated. Giemsa-stained buffy coat smears were prepared and revealed a few macrophages containing oval, nonflagellated protozoan forms, about 2 to 3 μm long (Fig. 15.1). A large nucleus, a small kinetoplast, and an axoneme were visible in several parasites.

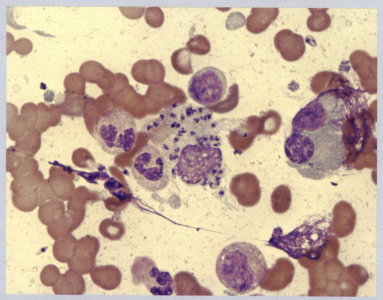

Figure 15.1

QUESTIONS

1. Which infection does this patient have? What is the name of the hemoflagellate which is causing his infection?

2. Name the three species belonging to this complex. In which parts of the world are these species located?

3. Which vectors are responsible for the transmission of this infection?

4. List four forms of infection caused by this genus of hemoflagellates. How does this patient's infection differ from the other three?

5. How is the diagnosis of this infection made?

6. What is the significance of the time of day (midnight) at which the patient was seen in the emergency department?

7. What causes the enlargement of the liver and spleen?

8. What causes the anemia and leukopenia characteristic of this infection?

9. Which complication may occur in this infection?

10. How is this infection treated?

ANSWERS

1. The patient has Old World visceral leishmaniasis, or kala-azar. Kala-azar, which means "black fever" in Hindi, refers to the characteristic darkening of the skin, not always apparent, which occurs mostly on the forehead, over the temples, and around the mouth. The hemoflagellate causing his illness is a member of the *Leishmania donovani* complex.

2. The three species belonging to the *L. donovani* complex include *L. donovani*, *L. infantum,* and *L. chagasi. L. donovani* occurs in Africa and Asia. *L. infantum* is found in Europe, Africa, the Mediterranean area, and southwestern Asia. *L. chagasi* is found primarily in Central and South America.

3. Sand flies in the genus *Phlebotomus* are vectors for most hemoflagellates in the *L. donovani* complex (*L. donovani* and *L. infantum*). Sand flies in the genus *Lutzomyia* are vectors for *L. chagasi.*

4. Parasites in the genus *Leishmania* cause not only visceral leishmaniasis (kala-azar) but also mucocutaneous leishmaniasis, Old World cutaneous leishmaniasis (oriental sore), and New World cutaneous leishmaniasis.

   Unlike cutaneous and mucocutaneous leishmaniasis, the parasites causing kala-azar may be found throughout the body. *L. donovani* does not usually cause skin lesions, other than a small papule at the insect bite. However, a condition known as dermal leishmanoid, characterized by the development of erythematous or depigmented macules, may occur in patients following treatment for visceral leishmaniasis. Although parasites causing cutaneous and mucocutaneous leishmaniasis are usually confined to the reticuloendothelial cells of the subcutaneous tissues and mucous membranes, visceral disease does occasionally occur, especially when underlying immunosuppressive disease exists, such as that associated with human immunodeficiency virus infections.

5. In areas where *Leishmania* is endemic, the diagnosis of visceral leishmaniasis is often based on clinical symptoms. Splenic aspirates are the preferred specimens for the recovery of *Leishmania* parasites. However, this invasive procedure poses a risk to the patient. Buffy coat preparations are recommended to spare the patient an invasive splenic biopsy, although buffy coat monocytes may not contain numerous organisms in many patients. Other specimens include liver biopsy samples, lymph node aspirates, and bone marrow aspirates.

The amastigotes may be detected in Giemsa-stained smears of tissues or clinical specimens. Amastigotes of *Trypanosoma cruzi* are indistinguishable from those found in leishmaniasis. Although culture and animal inoculation methods may be useful, these procedures are not available in most clinical microbiology laboratories.

Nucleic acid or antigen detection methods may also be used to make a diagnosis. PCR methods are quite sensitive and specific in diagnosing visceral leishmaniasis, as well as assessing response to treatment.

Serological methods are available for the diagnosis of visceral leishmaniasis, and newly developed assays show better sensitivity than older tests. However, these methods are not widely available. These tests include the enzyme-linked immunosorbent assay (ELISA), the direct agglutination test, an indirect fluorescent antibody assay (IFA), and a counterimmunoelectrophoresis assay. The Montenegro skin test is useful for epidemiological purposes in screening large populations in areas where *Leishmania* is endemic.

6. Apparently, there is a difference in the ease of detection of amastigotes in specimens collected during the day and at night. Saran et al. have reported that recovery of parasites is more common in specimens collected during the night.

7. Rapid proliferation of the cells of the reticuloendothelial system, including those in the liver and spleen, results in hypertrophy of these organs. The organs usually return to normal size following successful treatment.

8. Macrophages and monocytes parasitized by *Leishmania* protozoans rupture, leading to leukopenia. Hematopoiesis becomes depressed, with a shortened life span of red and white blood cells. Splenomegaly may result in increased destruction of erythrocytes and leukocytes, due to stasis of blood within the sinusoids.

9. Interstitial nephritis may develop as a complication of visceral leishmaniasis, with infiltration of lymphocytes and plasma cells. Rare ocular complications include keratitis, uveitis, retinal hemorrhage, iritis, and papillitis.

10. Patients, especially those who are malnourished or debilitated, should receive supportive care. Pentavalent antimony compounds have long been used for treating visceral leishmaniasis; however, treatment failures have been reported. Some cases of leishmaniasis have been successfully treated with liposomal amphotericin B. Therapy with paromomycin and allopurinol in combination with pentavalent antimonials has also proven effective.

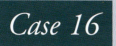

Case 16

A 17-year-old girl, who had never traveled outside the United States, had recently spent the summer working as a waitress in Nantucket, Mass. She had been previously healthy, although she had had a splenectomy due to injuries suffered in a ski accident. On her return to her home in Washington, D.C., she developed a headache, fatigue, fever, shaking chills, joint and muscle aches, and other vague flu-like symptoms, which persisted for a month. At that point, she visited her family doctor for medical advice.

The patient's physician ordered laboratory tests, including a blood count, and thick and thin blood smears. The thin smears, stained with Giemsa stain, revealed intraerythrocytic, pleomorphic, ringlike and crucifix-shaped structures, found peripherally in the pale red blood cells. Typical parasites are shown in Fig. 16.1.

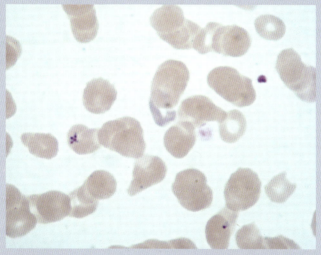

Figure 16.1

QUESTIONS

1. What is the probable diagnosis of this patient's infection? Name the protozoan blood parasite which is most likely to be responsible for this infection.

2. What are the ringlike and crucifix-shaped structures seen in the peripheral blood smear? Which aspect of the patient's history led to your conclusion about her diagnosis? Do you think that her history of having a splenectomy would have any relationship to her illness?

3. Why is this infection common only in certain geographical areas?

4. Which other infections are transmitted by the same vector?

5. Describe the life cycle of this parasite.

6. In which other manner may this infection be transmitted?

7. How do infections with this parasite in other geographical areas differ from the case described here?

8. How may this infection be treated?

ANSWERS

1. This patient had babesiosis. Although there are many species of *Babesia*, most human infections in the United States are caused by the blood parasite *Babesia microti*.

2. The intraerythrocytic ringlike structures seen in the thin smear resemble early trophozoite forms of species of *Plasmodium* (especially *Plasmodium falciparum*), which causes malaria. The ring form of *Plasmodium* and *Babesia* species consists of light blue cytoplasm and a pink to red nucleus. Although malaria is probably the best known parasitic bloodstream infection and might be expected to cause the symptoms found in this patient, the patient's lack of travel outside of the United States makes this diagnosis unlikely.

It is necessary to distinguish *Babesia* from *Plasmodium*. *Babesia* may be identified by the presence of a tetrad formation of chromatin, resembling a crucifix and known as a "Maltese cross" (Fig. 16.1), although this structure is not always present or is difficult to find. More commonly, wispy rings of different morphologies are observed. Other similarities between *Babesia* and *Plasmodium* include the appearance of appliqué forms and the presence of multiple ring forms per red blood cell. However, the absence of growing trophozoites and gametocytes in *Babesia* may be used to distinguish between the two protozoans. *Babesia* also lacks the pigment, hemozoin, found in erythrocytes infected by malarial parasites. Although diagnostic methods for babesiosis are also used to diagnose malaria, the former parasites, unlike malaria parasites, may be present in the blood at any time of day. As with malaria, blood smears should be prepared every 6 to 8 h for up to 3 days to rule out infection.

The patient had spent time in Nantucket. Babesiosis has most often been found in areas in the northeastern part of the United States, particularly in southern New England, Long Island, and the islands off the New England coast (Nantucket, Block Island, and Martha's Vineyard). However, babesiosis has also been found in other areas of the country, including Missouri, Georgia, and Wisconsin.

Although babesiosis has been associated with patients with a history of having a splenectomy, the closest association of splenectomy is with the cattle-associated *B. divergens* in Europe. Although there is no clear association of splenectomy with *B. microti* infection in the United States, disease is known to be more severe in splenectomized patients.

3. *B. microti* is transmitted by ticks of the genus *Ixodes*, which are commonly present in many geographical areas in the United States. Their widespread distribution may be because many animals in this country serve as reservoir hosts for these ticks.

4. *Borrelia burgdorferi*, the causative agent of Lyme disease, and *Ehrlichia* species, the cause of human granulocytic ehrlichiosis, are also transmitted by the *Ixodes* tick. The incidence of babesiosis has increased in recent years and appears to parallel the increase in the incidence of Lyme disease. Coinfection with *B. microti* and *Borrelia burgdorferi* has been reported and is associated with an illness which is more severe than either one alone.

5. Infective forms of *B. microti* are acquired by the larval or nymphal tick from the white-footed mouse. Sexual reproduction takes place in the tick. Vertical transmission of infection may also occur in ticks. Human infection occurs by the introduction of infective forms of the parasite into the bite wound while the tick is taking a blood meal.

6. Babesiosis is known to have been transmitted from asymptomatic blood donors to recipients during a blood transfusion.

7. Infections with *Babesia* differ in California and Europe from the case described here in the northeastern United States, where the infection is usually mild or subclinical. In these other areas, infections are often fulminant, causing a hemolytic disease in immunocompromised individuals. Splenectomized individuals are at particular risk of acquiring severe infections.

8. A combination of clindamycin and oral quinine is considered to be standard therapy to treat patients with babesiosis. An alternative regimen is a combination of azithromycin and either quinine or atovaquone.

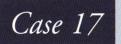

Case 17
A 37-year-old man with AIDS had been suffering from headache, fever, and fatigue for several weeks. He also had a history of seizures. He was brought to his family physician by his roommate. The roommate reported that the patient had been disoriented and confused for several weeks. The patient's CD4 T-lymphocyte count was determined to be 50/mm³.

Serological tests for *Toxoplasma*-specific immunoglobulin G were negative. A computed tomogram revealed multiple cerebral lesions. Histological methods were used to make a diagnosis (Fig. 17.1). After being treated with a combination of pyrimethamine and clarithromycin, the patient appeared to recover from his infection.

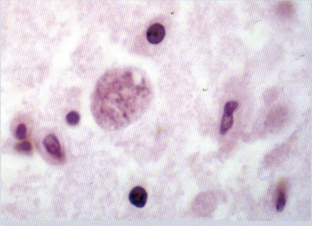

Figure 17.1

QUESTIONS

1. What is the likely diagnosis of this patient's parasitic illness?

2. What is the association between the patient's history of AIDS and this infection?

3. Which other group of individuals is at risk when infected with this parasite?

4. How is this infection transmitted?

5. Why was serology negative for this patient? How is the diagnosis of this illness made for immunocompromised patients including AIDS patients, transplant recipients, and patients with cancers or autoimmune diseases?

6. Describe the life cycle of this parasite.

7. What effect have the new antiretroviral therapies for AIDS (known as highly active antiretroviral therapy [HAART]) had on the frequency of this infection?

8. How might this patient be treated?

ANSWERS

1. The patient most probably has cerebral toxoplasmosis due to the coccidian protozoan parasite *Toxoplasma gondii*.

2. Most patients with toxoplasmosis are asymptomatic or have mild symptoms, similar to those of infectious mononucleosis, such as fever, chills, headache, muscle aches, and fatigue. However, in immunosuppressed individuals, such as those with AIDS, or otherwise compromised hosts, the infection may be severe, with neurological symptoms including encephalopathy, meningoencephalitis, and cerebral mass lesions. This complication is usually due to reactivation of a latent infection acquired before the development of AIDS rather than to primary infection with the parasite. Disseminated toxoplasmosis, with involvement of many organs, may occur.

3. Pregnant women who develop toxoplasmosis, particularly during the first 2 trimesters of pregnancy, are at risk of transmitting the infection across the placenta, resulting in severe tissue damage in their fetuses. Complications of congenital toxoplasmosis include malformation, abortion, or death of the newborn. In symptomatic pregnant women, chemotherapy may be administered to prevent congenital disease.

4. Human infection with *T. gondii* is usually acquired through accidental ingestion of infective tissue cysts in contaminated food such as raw or undercooked meat. Contact with oocyst-contaminated cat feces in a litter box may also transmit the infection. Contaminated soil may also be a source of disease. Although indoor cats fed with commercially prepared cat food are unlikely to harbor infective oocysts of *T. gondii*, outdoor cats, cats fed with uncooked food, or cats that hunt birds and other animals, which may act as reservoirs containing tissue cysts, are more likely to be infected.

Transmission of tachyzoites of *T. gondii* in transfused blood has been reported. Infection has also been acquired by transplantation of infected organs. Disease may result from reactivation of a latent infection or may be an acute primary infection.

5. Although the diagnosis of toxoplasmosis may be made serologically, interpretation of the results may be difficult. The detection of immunoglobulin G confirms only chronic infection and may be absent in AIDS patients with toxoplasmic encephalitis. In the absence of serological evidence of acute infection, histological or cytological demonstration of the organism replicating in tissue or identification of parasite-specific nucleic acid in CSF or bronchoalveolar lavage fluid may provide a diagnosis.

6. The life cycle of *T. gondii* is completed in the definitive feline host, most importantly the house cat. Cats become infected when they swallow infective oocysts, the resistant stages which contain sporozoites. Sporozoites invade and multiply in intestinal cells. The parasite produces schizonts and sexual stages (gametocytes) in the epithelial cells of the cat's small intestine. Fertilization occurs, and oocysts develop and are passed in the feces. These oocysts are unsporulated and become infective in about 2 days. Each oocyst contains one sporoblast. Development of infective sporozoites depends on environmental conditions.

In the human, multiplication occurs in the intestinal cells, but instead of sexual stages being produced, dissemination often occurs, with resistant stages forming in brain and muscle tissue. The trophozoites of *T. gondii* include the rapidly multiplying tachyzoites and the slower-multiplying bradyzoites, which form cysts in tissue. The organisms are obligate intracellular parasites in humans. Crescent-shaped tachyzoites are found in the early, acute stage of infection, while cysts containing bradyzoites are found predominantly in brain and muscle tissue, possibly due in part to the immune response of the host.

7. Encephalitis as a complication of toxoplasmosis was the most frequent CNS opportunistic infection in AIDS patients prior to the use of the new antiretroviral therapies for AIDS (known as HAART). These highly active agents have greatly reduced the occurrence of these infections in this population. It is recommended that all human immunodeficiency virus-infected persons be tested for *Toxoplasma*-specific antibodies soon after diagnosis to detect latent infection.

8. Although a combination of pyrimethamine and a sulfonamide is the standard regimen for treating *Toxoplasma* encephalitis in AIDS patients, intravenous clindamycin has also been used successfully. The use of oral clindamycin and pyrimethamine is also effective.

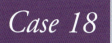

Case 18

A 35-year-old male medical student from Kenya, who was studying in the United States, presented to a hospital emergency room in Boston, Mass., after a trip home to visit relatives. His symptoms consisted of nausea, vomiting, fever, malaise, night sweats, and severe shaking chills. These symptoms had persisted for several weeks. Chills and fever occurred periodically, usually at 36- to 48-h intervals. An enlarged spleen was detected on physical examination. Blood was drawn for laboratory tests, including a platelet count, a complete blood count (CBC), and thick and thin blood smears.

The results of the CBC revealed that the patient was anemic (hemoglobin, 9.0 g/dl) and thrombocytopenic (platelets, 30,000/μl). Thick and thin smears were prepared and stained using the Giemsa method. Microscopic examination of these films revealed the presence of a large number (average of three parasites per oil immersion field) of intraerythrocytic parasitic forms, mostly in the shape of small rings (Fig. 18.1). A few cells contained multiple rings. A rare banana-shaped gametocyte was seen (Fig. 18.2). Some early ring trophozoites were identified as appliqué forms. Several blue rings with two red chromatin dots were seen. A small number of irregular dark bluish red dots were also seen in the erythrocytes. The red blood cells were normal in size and exhibited no stippling. Based on these findings, a diagnosis of infection with a blood parasite was made.

QUESTIONS

1. Which infection does this patient have? Which parasite is infecting him?

2. Describe the typical appearance of this parasite in thick and thin Giemsa-stained smears. What are the "red dots" seen in the smear?

3. What are the "appliqué" forms seen in the blood smear?

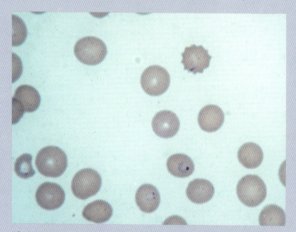

Figure 18.1

4. Describe the clinical illness caused by this parasite. Explain the severity of symptoms in this patient.

5. Why is infection by this species considered to be more serious than infection caused by other species?

6. Describe the life cycle of this parasite.

7. In addition to thick and thin blood smears, which other laboratory techniques are available to diagnose this infection?

8. How would this infection be treated?

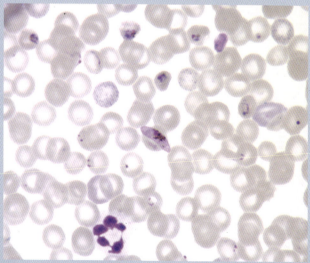

Figure 18.2

ANSWERS

1. The patient has malaria due to infection with *Plasmodium falciparum*.

2. The typical appearance of *P. falciparum* in peripheral blood usually includes only small, delicate ring forms in normal-sized and nonstippled erythrocytes, as was seen in this patient. The ring form of *Plasmodium* species consists of a light blue cytoplasm and a pink to red nucleus. Multiple rings may be observed in *P. falciparum*. Two dots of chromatin may be present on the ring forms. Although these asexual stages are very small, they can be readily recognized in thick films. Early ring stage forms of the four species of *Plasmodium* are morphologically similar. Parasitemia with *P. falciparum* may be high. Schüffner's dots are absent. Crescent-shaped or banana-shaped gametocytes are occasionally seen in late infections with *P. falciparum*. Mature schizonts are generally not seen in peripheral blood, except in particularly severe cases of infection.

The red dots seen in the Giemsa-stained smear are Maurer's dots. Although these dots may be seen in infections caused by *P. falciparum*, they are not common and are not a reliable diagnostic characteristic.

3. The appliqué (also called accolé) forms are early ring-stage trophozoites of *P. falciparum*, found at the periphery of red blood cells.

4. *P. falciparum* causes malignant tertian malaria, which is characterized by cycles and paroxysms every 36 to 48 h. Symptoms of infection with this species of *Plasmodium* are usually more severe than symptoms of infection with other species. This type of malaria is common and occurs worldwide.

P. falciparum attacks both young and old erythrocytes, usually resulting in heavy infection. However, severe cases of malaria, including cerebral malaria, may occur if even a small number of parasites are present. This type of illness tends to occur in patients from the United States not previously exposed to this parasite. These individuals travel outside the country and become infected with *P. falciparum*. Since these patients lack antibodies from previous exposures, they tend to be symptomatic early in the course of infection and have a low parasitemia when they present to their physicians. Relapse of infection with this parasite does not occur.

This patient had just returned from a visit to Kenya. His immunity had probably declined during his stay in the United States. When he became infected during his vacation, he developed severe symptoms more quickly than if his immunity had been optimal.

5. The large number of parasites may result in tissue hypoxia and disseminated intravascular coagulation. Infections caused by *P. falciparum* may lead to severe, often fulminant illness, with the development of acute tubular necrosis and renal failure and with CNS involvement (cerebral malaria), characterized by altered mental status and coma.

Blackwater fever is a rare complication of malaria, usually *P. falciparum* malaria. Massive intravascular hemolysis causes hemoglobinuria, with a blackening of the urine due to a high methemoglobin level in the urine. This illness usually begins during a paroxysm of falciparum malaria but may occur in the absence of symptoms. The massive destruction of red blood cells may lead to severe anemia.

6. The malarial life cycle involves two hosts, a definitive host and an intermediate host. Asexual reproduction (schizogony) occurs in the human host. The life cycle begins when, during a blood meal, sporozoites from a malaria-infected female anopheline mosquito (definitive host) are inoculated into the bloodstream of a human host. The exoerythrocytic stage is initiated when sporozoites leave the blood and travel to the liver. They invade hepatic parenchymal cells, forming schizonts. The patient remains asymptomatic at this time. The schizonts mature and rupture, releasing many merozoites into the bloodstream, where they invade erythrocytes, beginning the erythrocytic cycle.

Asexual reproduction (schizogony) occurs in the erythrocytes. The merozoite lies within a vacuole within the red blood cell and digests hemoglobin by the action of proteases. The ring-stage trophozoites mature into schizonts, which rupture, releasing many merozoites and precipitating clinical symptoms. Merozoites begin a new cycle by entering more erythrocytes. Eventually, after a few erythrocytic generations, the merozoites differentiate into sexual male and female gametocytes, which are picked up by a feeding mosquito.

Sexual reproduction (sporogony) occurs in the mosquito. A female anopheline mosquito ingests malarial macrogametocytes (female) and microgametocytes (male) when it feeds on an infected individual. These quickly develop into gametes in the mosquito gut. Fertilization occurs when a microgamete penetrates a macrogamete, with the formation of a zygote, which puts out a pseudopod and becomes elongated. This motile form is called an ookinete. The ookinete develops into a spherical oocyst in the gut wall of the insect. Sporozoites develop within the oocyst. The oocyst ruptures, with the release of numerous sporozoites, which travel to the salivary glands of the insect. Inoculation of the sporozoites into another human host begins the life cycle again.

7. Alternative approaches to the diagnosis of malaria include detection of *Plasmodium* DNA by using the acridine orange stain on buffy coat smears, PCR methods, and detection of *Plasmodium* antigens in circulating blood. Malaria has also been diagnosed by the demonstration of unexpected abnormalities with an automated hematology analyzer.

8. A variety of drugs are available to treat malaria, and their use is based on their effects on the parasite at various stages of the life cycle. Patients with malaria are often treated with chloroquine. However, some strains of *P. falciparum* are resistant to this agent. Because of this and because of advances in the treatment of serious complications of this infection, therapy for these cases may be complex. Mefloquine is an effective drug which may be used to treat chloroquine-resistant *P. falciparum,* both therapeutically and prophylactically, although resistance has been reported. Neurological and neuropsychiatric side effects may occur with this agent. Combinations of doxycycline or clindamycin plus quinine may be considered as alternative agents for the treatment of drug-resistant falciparum malaria.

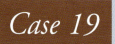

Case 19

A 39-year-old woman who had been diagnosed with AIDS visited the emergency department complaining of severe headache, fever, vomiting, and nausea of several weeks' duration. A lumbar puncture was performed, and CSF was collected and sent to the laboratory for analysis. A Gram stain showed many white blood cells but no bacteria. Bacterial and viral cultures were negative.

Neuroimaging studies were suggestive of meningoencephalitis. GAE was suspected. At the suggestion of an infectious-disease consultant, a CSF specimen was collected and sent to a reference laboratory for tissue culture. Trophozoites of a leptomyxid ameba, having broad fingerlike pseudopodia, were isolated. Electron microscopy and histochemical studies were used to confirm the diagnosis. Figure 19.1 shows trophozoites of this parasite in brain tissue.

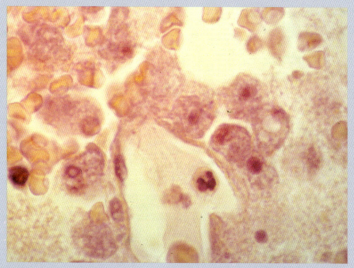

Figure 19.1

QUESTIONS

1. What is the name of the leptomyxid ameba causing GAE in this patient?

2. How does this infection compare with GAE caused by another free-living ameba?

3. How do the trophozoites and cysts of these two amebae differ?

4. How does this infection differ from PAM? How is this patient's history relevant to her infection?

5. How do the life cycles of *Acanthamoeba, Balamuthia mandrillaris,* and *Naegleria fowleri* differ?

6. How can a definitive identification of this ameba be made?

7. How do the pathologies of *Balamuthia* and *Acanthamoeba* differ?

8. How is this infection treated?

ANSWERS

1. The relatively uncommon free-living ameba causing this patient's infection is *Balamuthia mandrillaris*. This parasite, only recently recognized, was once thought to be nonpathogenic in humans but is now known to cause GAE, an infection similar to that caused by *Acanthamoeba*. *B. mandrillaris* has recently joined *Acanthamoeba* in the family Acanthamoebidae.

2. This infection is quite similar to GAE caused by *Acanthamoeba*. Although the portal of entry is not known for certain, it is likely that, as with *Acanthamoeba,* the parasite enters the host through the nostrils, by way of the lower respiratory tract, or through breaks in the skin, with hematogenous spread. The clinical course of the infection is subacute or chronic, as seen in *Acanthamoeba* infections. The incubation period is unknown. It is difficult to distinguish *Acanthamoeba* and *B. mandrillaris* by light microscopy alone.

3. Like *Acanthamoeba*, *B. mandrillaris* does not have a flagellated stage in its life cycle, only a trophozoite and a cyst stage. The trophozoites of *B. mandrillaris* are irregular in shape, measure 12 to 60 μm in diameter (average, 30 μm), and show broad pseudopodia and extensive branching in culture. As the tissue cells are destroyed, fingerlike pseudopodia develop. The trophozoites usually have one nucleus (occasionally two), with a central karyosome. The motile trophozoites of *Acanthamoeba* have spinelike pseudopods. The spherical cysts of *B. mandrillaris* measure 6 to 30 μm and have a double wall. The outer wall is thick and irregular. *Acanthamoeba* cysts are round and are also characterized by having a double wall, with the outer wall being slightly wrinkled. Both *Acanthamoeba* and *B. mandrillaris* possess a multilayered microtubule-organizing center.

4. PAM, caused by the free-living ameba *N. fowleri,* is a rare and rapidly progressive, fatal illness in healthy children and young adults, who have a history of swimming or diving in local water sources in warm weather. GAE caused by *B. mandrillaris* is a less acute and fulminant infection than PAM. It is an opportunistic infection seen primarily in immunocompromised patients. However, a recently reported case of fatal meningoencephalitis in a child was linked to an environmental source (potted soil).

   Trophozoites of *N. fowleri* may be found in freshwater sources, including lakes, ponds, streams, hot springs, irrigation ditches, and swimming pools. However, there is no association of GAE with a history of swimming in fresh water. This patient was at risk for infection due to her immunocompromised status.

5. There are three stages in the life cycle of *N. fowleri,* including both ameboid and flagellate stages. These stages include an amebic trophozoite, a flagellated form possessing two flagella, and a resistant cyst stage. *Acanthamoeba* and *B. mandrillaris* lack the flagellate stage. In *Acanthamoeba* infections, both trophozoites and cysts are found in tissues, while in infections with *N. fowleri,* only trophozoites are found.

6. To definitively identify *B. mandrillaris*, electron microscopy and histochemical methods must be employed. Unlike *Acanthamoeba* and *N. fowleri*, this ameba cannot be grown in culture with bacteria as a nutrient source. However, it may be isolated by using a tissue culture monolayer or an enriched, cell-free medium.

7. *Balamuthia* causes inflammation, multiple necrotic foci, and cerebral edema. *Acanthamoeba* causes focal necrosis and the development of granulomas.

8. Although in vitro studies indicate that *B. mandrillaris* is susceptible to pentamidine isethionate and that infected patients may benefit from this treatment, there have been no documented reports of recovery from this infection.

Case 20

A 29-year-old woman presented to the emergency department complaining of severe eye pain and a recent loss of vision in her right eye over the past few weeks. She had no previous eye problems, although she had worn contact lenses since the age of 20. Her practice was to prepare her own saline solution, using tap water, to clean her lenses.

The examination of her eye revealed a corneal ulcer. Based on her history and a suspicion that the patient might have an amebic infection, a corneal biopsy specimen was sent to the pathology laboratory for analysis. The slide prepared from the specimen showed amebic trophozoites. Histological preparations revealed numerous neutrophils and monocytes. Cultures were negative for bacteria and viruses. An amebic parasite was recovered in culture.

QUESTIONS

1. Which ameba would you expect to be causing this patient's infection?

2. Why might this infection be difficult to diagnose microscopically?

3. Which misdiagnosis is common in these infections?

4. How does the laboratory culture this parasite?

5. Which cytological techniques are available for the diagnosis of this infection?

6. Which risk factor did this patient have?

7. How is this infection treated?

8. How may this infection be prevented?

9. Which serious complication may occur as a result of this infection?

ANSWERS

1. An *Acanthamoeba* sp. is the ameba causing this woman's painful ocular infection, known as *Acanthamoeba* keratitis.

2. The recognition of *Acanthamoeba* trophozoites in ocular specimens is difficult. Although histological examination of corneal tissue may reveal this parasite, trophozoites may easily be confused with neutrophils and monocytes, which were found in histological preparations of this patient's specimen. Tissue stains, such as Gomori's silver stain, Calcofluor White, and the periodic acid-Schiff stain, may be used to detect cysts.

3. Ocular infections with *Acanthamoeba* spp. can resemble infections caused by bacteria such as *Pseudomonas aeruginosa,* fungi, and viruses. Herpes simplex virus causes a keratitis that is most often confused with this infection. However, this viral infection is rarely associated with the severe pain which accompanies *Acanthamoeba* keratitis.

4. The amebae may be cultured by seeding agar plates with bacterial cells of *Escherichia coli,* which serve as nutrients, before inoculating the media with corneal scrapings from the patient. The agar plates are incubated at 37°C and examined daily for the telltale tracks which are seen in areas of bacterial growth. *Acanthamoeba* spp. have been cultured from contact lenses and lens-cleaning solutions when corneal scrapings have been negative.

5. A cytological diagnosis may be made by employing various staining techniques. An indirect immunofluorescence method has been used in the detection of amebic cysts in corneal scrapings. Calcofluor White has also been effective in demonstrating amebic cysts, which stain a bright apple green with this chemofluorescent dye.

6. The greatest risk factor for developing *Acanthamoeba* keratitis is the use of homemade or commercial solutions that have been contaminated during use or the use of an outdated product as a cleansing agent for contact lenses. This infection has increased in the United States in recent years, mainly due to the heightened popularity of newer types of contact lenses. Disinfecting solutions used for soft lenses do not always kill the organisms. Apparently, the risk for acquiring *Acanthamoeba* keratitis is not related to the type of lens material used. The trophozoites of *Acanthamoeba* spp. proliferate on the contact lens and are transferred to the corneal epithelium of the eye when the lens is inserted.

7. Earlier cases of *Acanthamoeba* keratitis required corneal transplants to control the infection. Today, antiamebic agents are available to treat the infection. Propamidine is the drug of choice to treat *Acanthamoeba* keratitis. Other agents include ketoconazole, miconazole, pentamidine isethionate, and rifampin. Combination therapy is often effective. However, sight may be lost even when appropriate therapy is used. Bacterial superinfections may also occur.

8. *Acanthamoeba* keratitis can be prevented by careful attention to the care and cleansing of contact lenses. Tap water should not be used to prepare cleansing solutions or to rinse contact lenses. The manufacturer's recommendations should be followed, and outdated products should never be used.

9. The patient may suffer permanent impairment of vision and blindness in the infected eye, and a corneal transplant may be required.

Case 21

A 25-year-old woman had recently returned to the United States from a 2-week safari vacation in Tanzania. She visited several game parks during her stay in Africa. The patient presented to the emergency room complaining of headache, anorexia, diarrhea, vomiting, chills, fever, night sweats, and increasing sleepiness. She reported having received many bug bites during her trip to the game parks. Physical examination revealed a pale, emaciated woman with a painless, erythematous lesion located on her shoulder. No adenopathy was noted.

Blood was drawn for laboratory studies. Results indicated a systemic inflammatory response. The C-reactive protein level was high at 210 mg/liter. Thrombocytopenia was noted, with a platelet count of $75 \times 10^3/\mu l$. The patient was anemic, with a hemoglobin count of 8.5 g/dl. Thick and thin blood smears were prepared and stained using the Giemsa method. A large number of pleomorphic hemoflagellates, some being slender and some being stumpy, were visible in the blood smears. Typical parasites are shown in Fig. 21.1.

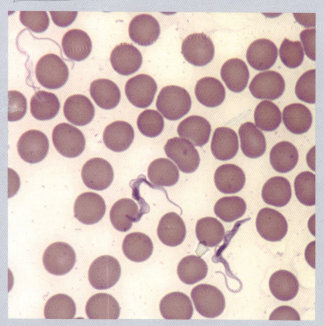

Figure 21.1

QUESTIONS

1. Which infection does this patient have? What is the name of the hemoflagellate causing her infection?

2. What is the name of the erythematous lesion noted on the patient's shoulder?

3. What is the association of this illness with the patient's visits to East African game parks? Why is the history of insect bites relevant to the patient's illness?

4. Which group of insects is important vectors of this infection?

5. Why is infection caused by this hemoflagellate subspecies considered to be more serious than infection caused by other subspecies?

6. How is this infection treated?

7. What is the disadvantage of using blood smears to diagnose this infection? Are nonhematological methods available to make the diagnosis?

ANSWERS

1. The patient has East African trypanosomiasis (African sleeping sickness) caused by the hemoflagellate *Trypanosoma brucei rhodesiense*.

2. The painful, indurated, erythematous lesion, more common in non-Africans, is known as a trypanosomal chancre.

3. Many of the animals which the safari tourist will see, including waterbucks, oxen, and lions, are bitten by game-feeding tsetse flies and are therefore potential reservoirs for infection with the trypanosomes that cause East African trypanosomiasis. Unlike West African trypanosomiasis (caused by *T. brucei gambiense*), where the human population remains the most important reservoir, wild and domestic animals are important reservoirs for *T. brucei rhodesiense*.

4. It has been postulated that the hemoflagellates were originally insect parasites. Tsetse flies in the *Glossina morsitans* group are important vectors for transmission of *T. brucei rhodesiense*, while *G. palpalis* tsetse flies are more important in the transmission of *T. brucei gambiense*.

5. Infection with *T. brucei rhodesiense* is considered more serious than infection with *T. brucei gambiense* due to the short incubation period and the fulminant nature of the former infection. *T. brucei gambiense* causes a chronic illness with a slow, mild clinical course, while infection with *T. brucei rhodesiense* results in an acute illness with rapid progression (in as little as 1 month) to fatal CNS disease. Patients may die before symptoms of disease indicate the severity of this infection. The trypomastigotes of *T. brucei gambiense* and *T. brucei rhodesiense* are morphologically identical. It is important to elicit the patient's travel history to make a correct diagnosis.

6. Treatment of trypanosomiasis includes pentamidine isethionate, which does not pass the blood-brain barrier, and intravenous suramin. However, treatment is usually effective only during the early stages of disease. Transient proteinuria is a known side effect of suramin treatment. CNS involvement occurring during late-stage Gambian and Rhodesian sleeping sickness may be treated with melarsoprol, although toxic side effects are frequently associated with this agent.

7. Although trypomastigotes are usually found in large numbers in the blood during febrile periods, only small numbers are present during afebrile periods. Trypomastigotes are better demonstrated in CSF during later stages of disease.

   In addition to blood smears, other methods are available to diagnose trypanosomiasis. Serological assays available include latex agglutination tests and immunofluorescence assays. Other diagnostic tests include an enzyme-linked immunosorbent assay (ELISA) used to detect antigen in serum and CSF. An agglutination assay called the card agglutination trypanosomiasis test is commercially available for screening purposes and epidemiological surveys. PCR is also available. Although culture on specialized media is possible, these methods are not suitable for routine clinical laboratories.

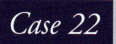

Case 22

A previously healthy 22-year-old woman returned to Boston after a vacation in Kenya. Two weeks later, she visited a local emergency room for treatment of multiple ulcerated skin lesions on her face and extremities. An aspirate taken from beneath an ulcer bed was sent to the laboratory for examination. A Giemsa-stained smear showed monocytes containing small, oval, nonmotile parasitic forms measuring 2 to 3 μm in length. Amastigotes characteristic for this parasite are shown in Fig. 22.1.

A skin test was performed and was strongly positive for a hemoflagellate infection.

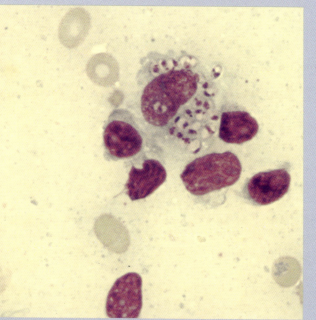

Figure 22.1

QUESTIONS

1. Which infection does this patient have? What is the name of the hemoflagellate causing her infection?

2. Name the three species belonging to this complex.

3. Which vector is responsible for the transmission of this infection?

4. Which stage of this parasite is the infective form?

5. Which stage of this parasite is seen in human blood smears?

6. What is the skin test used on the patient? How is this test useful in screening the population in areas of endemic infection?

7. Which treatment is recommended for this infection?

8. How is the diagnosis of this infection made?

ANSWERS

1. The patient has Old World cutaneous leishmaniasis, or Oriental sore. The hemoflagellate causing her illness is a member of the *Leishmania tropica* complex.

2. The three species belonging to the *L. tropica* complex include *L. tropica*, *L. major*, and *L. aethiopica*.

3. The *Phlebotomus* sand fly is the vector for hemoflagellates in the *L. tropica* complex.

4. The promastigote, which is an elongated, motile, extracellular stage, is the infective form of the *Leishmania* parasite. This form is injected into the skin of a human while a phlebotomine fly is taking a blood meal.

5. The amastigote stage, a small, nonmotile, intracellular form of the *Leishmania* parasite, is seen in human blood smears.

6. The Montenegro (leishmanin) skin test, involving the intradermal injection of a suspension of killed promastigotes, was the skin test used on this patient. This test is useful in screening large populations at risk of developing leishmaniasis.

7. Most patients with Old World cutaneous leishmaniasis do not require treatment. Lesions usually heal in several months to a few years. Lesions on the face may be treated with pentavalent antimonials, such as antimony sodium gluconate (sodium stibogluconate), which is the drug of choice for the treatment of cutaneous leishmaniasis. An exception is the Ethiopian form of diffuse cutaneous leishmaniasis, which is reported to respond better to pentamidine. Intramuscular human gamma interferon has recently been added to the regimen of drugs used to treat this infection.

   Intradermal injections of gamma interferon around cutaneous lesions has been shown to be effective. It appears that the cell-mediated immune response elicited by the interferon aids in the healing of these ulcers. Chemotherapy should be given in adequate doses and for a sufficient period (often weeks to months) to effect a cure.

8. In areas where *Leishmania* is endemic, the diagnosis of cutaneous leishmaniasis is often based on clinical symptoms. The amastigotes may be detected in Giemsa-stained smears of biopsy materials, or the promastigotes may be grown in culture. In a patient such as this, with multiple lesions, specimens should be collected from the advancing margin of the ulcer in the more active or recent lesions. Tissue imprint or touch preparations are also suitable for diagnosis. Multiple slides should be examined.

   Serological techniques are not useful in diagnosing cutaneous leishmaniasis, since antibody detection is variable. Antibody titers may be too low to be detected, yielding false-negative reactions, and cross-reactions may occur, with false-positive results. As mentioned above, the Montenegro skin test is useful for epidemiological purposes in screening large populations in areas of endemic infection.

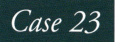

Case 23 A 45-year-old man was seen in the emergency department for persistent night sweats, headache, intermittent fever, and severe chills, which occurred approximately every 48 h. The patient was born in Asia and had moved to the United States 5 years earlier. At that time, he had suffered a similar illness, was treated, and appeared to make a good recovery. Blood was drawn for laboratory studies including a hemoglobin determination and thick and thin blood smears for parasites.

The patient was slightly anemic, with a hemoglobin level of 9.5 g/dl. Examination of Giemsa-stained blood films revealed the presence of enlarged red blood cells containing trophozoite forms (Fig. 23.1). Several irregular ameboid trophozoites containing brown granules were seen. Eosinophilic stippling was visible in the cytoplasm of the erythrocytes. A few round to oval gametocytes were seen. Based on these findings, a diagnosis of infection with a blood parasite was made.

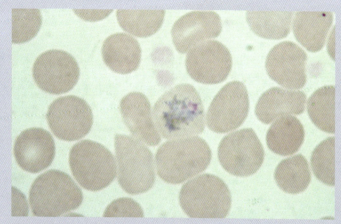

Figure 23.1

QUESTIONS

1. Which infection does this patient have? Which parasite is infecting him?

2. Describe the typical appearance of this parasite in thick and thin Giemsa-stained smears.

3. Which blood protozoan parasite morphologically resembles this parasite?

4. Comment on the size of the erythrocytes. What do we call the eosinophilic stippling seen in these cells? Which other species causes this characteristic?

5. Describe the clinical illness caused by this parasite. Which serious complication may occur with this infection?

6. How does the life cycle of different species of this parasite vary? How does this fact relate to this patient's infection?

7. How would this patient be treated?

ANSWERS

1. The patient has malaria caused by *Plasmodium vivax*.

2. In a patient infected with *P. vivax*, blood smears may reveal several stages during asexual development, as well as round to oval gametocytes, which are rarely seen, depending on when the blood is drawn during the cycle. Erythrocytes are enlarged. Delicate ring forms and ameboid trophozoites are common in these infections. A mature schizont contains approximately 12 to 24 merozoites, but the number tends to be around 16.

3. *P. ovale* is morphologically similar to *P. vivax*, although the rings of the former protozoan are smaller. The ring form of *Plasmodium* species consists of a light blue cytoplasm and a pink to red nucleus. Trophozoites of *P. ovale* are less ameboid than those of *P. vivax*. Early-ring-stage forms of the four species of *Plasmodium* are morphologically similar.

4. Erythrocytes infected with *P. vivax* are enlarged. This parasite infects young red blood cells, which are known as reticulocytes. The eosinophilic stippling is known as Schüffner's dots, which are present in most cells, excluding those harboring the early ring forms. They are also present in infections with *P. ovale* but not in those with *P. malariae* or *P. falciparum*.

5. *P. vivax* causes benign tertian malaria and is associated with moderate to severe symptoms, including chills and fever. The illness is characterized by cycles and paroxysms every 48 h. Although severe complications are rare with this infection, splenomegaly and, rarely, splenic rupture may occur.

6. This patient is suffering a relapse of his earlier malarial infection. Relapses of *P. vivax* infection occur after weeks, months, or up to 5 years or even longer.
   In patients infected with *P. vivax* and *P. ovale*, a proportion of the sporozoites infecting the hepatocytes apparently enter a resting phase before beginning asexual reproduction, while *P. falciparum* and *P. malariae* begin asexual reproduction immediately. The resting sporozoites are known as hypnozoites. Hypnozoites remain in a latent stage in the liver. After a variable period, the hypnozoites may become reactivated, leading to the relapses characteristic of *P. vivax* and, less commonly, *P. ovale* malarial infections. Since no persistent hypnozoites are associated with *P. falciparum* and *P. malariae*, relapses of infection with these parasites do not occur.

7. Therapy for malaria has become increasingly complex. A variety of drugs are available, and their use is based on their effects on the parasite at various stages of the life cycle. Although resistance of *P. falciparum* to chloroquine is well known, this drug is generally effective in treating infections with *P. vivax*, as well as *P. malariae* and *P. ovale*. However, there have been recent reports of chloroquine-resistant *P. vivax* infections in Indonesia and Oceania.

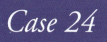

Case 24

A 25-year-old nurse had recently returned to the United States from a stay in Brazil, where she had worked at a clinic treating rural patients. She developed fever, anorexia, weight loss, shortness of breath, and myalgia and visited her primary care doctor. Physical examination revealed a thin woman with a slightly enlarged liver and spleen and with lymphadenopathy. She had upper and lower eyelid edema in her right eye, along with conjunctivitis. An electrocardiogram showed abnormalities of the P and T waves and the QRS complex, as well as cardiomegaly.

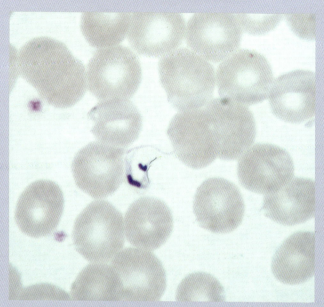

Thick and thin blood smears were ordered and were stained by the Giemsa method. Microscopic examination revealed a few flagellated spindle-shaped protozoan parasites (some assuming a C shape) with undulating membranes. A diagnosis of an infection with a blood parasite was made. A characteristic parasite is shown in Fig. 24.1.

Figure 24.1

QUESTIONS

chaga's disease

1. What is the name of this patient's illness? Which blood protozoan parasite is causing the infection? *T. cruzi*

2. How is this infection transmitted? *contact c contaminated feaces and urine of Reuvined bug ??*

3. Why is the vector for this protozoan known as the "kissing bug"?

4. Describe the life cycle of this parasite. *trypomastigotes - Amastigotes - trypomastigote*

5. What is the name of the lesion that may develop at the site of inoculation of *chagoma* the parasite? What is the name given to the unilateral edema of the eye in this disease? *Romana's Sign*

6. Which methods are available to diagnosis this infection? *- blood smear Serology*

7. How does this parasite differ from other parasites in the same genus?

8. How is this infection treated?

9. This infection may be acquired during blood transfusion. List other protozoan parasitic infections that may be transmitted during blood transfusions.

10. Explain the cardiac abnormalities found in this patient. Which other complication may occur? *Peri... ... ... cardiac failure myocarditis meningo encephalitis cardiomegaly*

ANSWERS

1. The patient has American trypanosomiasis, or Chagas' disease. This infection is caused by *Trypanosoma cruzi*.

2. *T. cruzi* is typically transmitted when an infected reduviid (triatomid) bug feeds on a human host. Transmission of Chagas' disease has also occurred during blood transfusions and organ transplantation, transplacentally, and occasionally by accidental ingestion of the insect vector.

3. The reduviid or triatomid bug, the vector for Chagas' disease, is called the kissing bug due to its tendency to bite the patient on the lips or face.

4. While feeding on a host, the triatomid bug releases metacyclic trypomastigotes in its feces. These infective forms are rubbed into the bite wound or pass through intact mucosal membranes such as the conjunctiva. In the human host, parasites penetrate and multiply in various cells, typically nucleated cells. Inside these cells, trypomastigotes transform into amastigotes, which multiply by binary fission and differentiate into trypomastigotes in infected tissues. On rupture of the cell, these forms are released into the bloodstream. Trypomastigotes continue to invade a variety of host tissue cells and transform into intracellular amastigotes.

Triatomid bugs ingest trypomastigotes while feeding on an infected human host. Ingested trypomastigotes transform into epimastigotes in the gut of the bug. Multiplication occurs in the midgut. Metacyclic trypomastigotes develop in the hindgut of the bug. The cycle continues when the bug releases these infective forms when feeding on its next human host.

5. A painful, erythematous, indurated local lesion called a chagoma may develop at the site of inoculation, most often on the face. This erythematous lesion is a result of an acute inflammatory reaction which blocks the flow of lymph. Trypomastigotes and amastigotes may be aspirated from chagomas during early stages of infection. The name given to the unilateral edema affecting the eyelids is Romaña's sign. The edema, which is often accompanied by conjunctivitis, may spread to the cheek and neck of the same side.

6. The trypomastigotes of *T. cruzi* are usually visible in thick or thin blood smears stained with Giemsa stain or in buffy coats in patients with acute Chagas' disease. They are not visible during the chronic phase of illness. The trypomastigote is typically C shaped, U shaped, or spindle shaped, with a large kinetoplast located in a posterior position. An undulating membrane extends along the organism and then extends beyond the body as a flagellum. Amastigotes of *T. cruzi* are indistinguishable from those found in leishmaniasis.

Antibody detection by serological methods is most useful in the diagnosis of chronic disease. Serological methods available include the complement fixation assay, the indirect hemagglutination assay, IFA, ELISA, the radioimmunoprecipitation assay, and latex agglutination. An ELISA procedure to detect *T. cruzi* antigen in urine has recently been described. Testing combinations used to diagnose Chagas' disease include the ELISA and IFA and the ELISA and IHA. These methods are also useful to screen blood donors in areas of endemic infection, such as South American countries, where Chagas' disease is a public health problem.

PCR methods for *T. cruzi* kinetoplast DNA detection are more sensitive and specific than traditional tests and are useful to diagnose acute and chronic Chagas' disease as well as to monitor therapy. This procedure, however, is not available in most clinical laboratories.

Xenodiagnosis is a technique whereby uninfected reduviid bugs bred in the laboratory are fed on the patient's blood. If parasites are present in the patient's blood, they multiply in the insect gut and may be recovered from the gut contents about 4 weeks later. *T. cruzi* may also be cultured in specialized media.

7. *T. cruzi* differs from other trypanosomes infecting humans by having, in addition to the trypomastigote form found in circulating blood, an intracellular amastigote form found in cardiac muscle and other tissues.

8. Most drugs have proven to be ineffective in treating Chagas' disease. Although acute Chagas' disease may be treated with nifurtimox, which is the drug of choice, this drug should not be used during pregnancy. Alternative drugs include allopurinol and benznidazole. No effective therapy is available to treat chronic disease. In late stages of disease, supportive care to relieve disease symptoms is advocated.

9. Other transfusion-transmitted protozoan infections include malaria, leishmaniasis, toxoplasmosis, and babesiosis.

10. EKG abnormalities are not infrequent findings in patients with Chagas' disease. Some patients show partial or complete atrioventricular block, right bundle branch block, or premature ventricular contractions, as well as abnormal P and T waves and QRS complex, as was seen in this patient. Progressive congestive heart failure may develop.

Dilatation of the digestive tract, including megaesophagus and megacolon, may occur, although it is less common than cardiac problems.

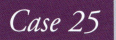

Case 25

A 29-year-old woman returning from a safari in tropical Africa was admitted to the hospital with a 1-month history of mild flu-like symptoms, including intermittent fever and chills (which occurred approximately every 48 h), headache, night sweats, diarrhea, and back and abdominal pain. When she was examined on admission, she had splenomegaly. Blood was drawn for laboratory tests, including a CBC, and thick and thin blood smears.

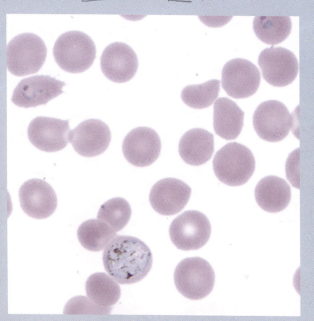

Figure 25.1

The patient was slightly anemic, with a hemoglobin level of 10 g/dl. Thick and thin blood smears were made and stained by the Giemsa method. Microscopic examination of the thin smear revealed enlarged, oval, pale erythrocytes, with fimbriated edges and containing distinct red Schüffner's dots. The parasite is shown in Fig. 25.1. Several slightly ameboid trophozoites and a very rare small gametocyte were also seen. Parasitemia was low, with no more than 1% infected red blood cells.

QUESTIONS

1. Which infection does this patient have? Which parasite is infecting her?

2. Describe the typical appearance of erythrocytes infected by this parasite in Giemsa-stained smears.

3. Which protozoan blood parasite morphologically resembles this parasite?

4. Describe the clinical illness caused by this parasite.

5. Why should thick and thin blood films be ordered to diagnose this illness? What are the advantages and disadvantages of each method?

6. How would this patient be treated?

ANSWERS

1. The patient has malaria caused by *Plasmodium ovale*.

2. *P. ovale* parasitizes reticulocytes (young erythrocytes). These cells are enlarged, with fimbriated edges, and may be oval. The eosinophilic stippling known as Schüffner's dots is present. These dots are very prominent when the stain is alkaline, as recommended.

3. *P. vivax* is morphologically similar to *P. ovale*, although the rings of the latter protozoan are smaller. The ring form of *Plasmodium* species consists of a light blue cytoplasm and a pink to red nucleus. Trophozoites of *P. ovale* are less ameboid than those of *P. vivax*. Early-ring-stage forms of the four species of *Plasmodium* are morphologically similar. A mature schizont contains 8 to 12 merozoites, but usually 8.

4. *P. ovale* causes tertian malaria, with mild symptoms, and is characterized by cycles and paroxysms every 48 h. Cerebral involvement may occur. Although not as common as in *P. vivax* malaria, relapses of *P. ovale* malaria may occur.

5. Both thick and thin films should be routinely used for the identification of malarial parasites. There are certain advantages and disadvantages to each method. The thick film is useful as a screening tool, while the thin film is preferred for a definitive diagnosis.

Advantages of thick blood films include the increased volume of blood examined. This increases the ability to detect light infections. Malaria pigment, as well as Schüffner's dots, may be visible at the periphery of the smear, where cells are not completely lysed. Disadvantages of thick blood films include the inability to compare the sizes of infected and uninfected erythrocytes because of hemolysis. Distortion of parasites may occur. It is difficult to identify the parasite to species level in thick films. Thick films often flake off during the staining process and may not stain properly if the film is too thick. Brief fixation of thick films in acetone after drying may improve the durability of these smears and enhance the adherence of blood to the slide. An additional disadvantage of thick smears is the fact that the ovoid and fimbriated appearance of the red blood cells characteristic of infection with *P. ovale* is not seen.

Thin films have the advantage of allowing visualization of red blood cell morphology, enhancing the ability to compare the sizes of infected and uninfected cells. It is easier to calculate the percentage of infected cells and to identify the parasite to species level in thin films. Thin films have the disadvantage of being less sensitive than thick films; low levels of parasites may be missed. Thin films must be carefully prepared to avoid poor smears as a result of having too much or too little blood.

It is imperative to use clean, grease-free glass slides with both methods to ensure proper smear preparation.

6. Therapy for malaria has become increasingly complex. A variety of drugs are available, and their use is based on their effects on the parasite at various stages of the life cycle Although resistance of *P. falciparum* to chloroquine is well known, this drug is generally effective in treating infections with *P. vivax, P. malariae,* and *P. ovale.*

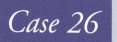

Case 26 A previously healthy 19-year-old woman, who had spent several months of the previous year as a student in Brazil, presented at an emergency department complaining of stuffy nose and painful ulcers on her lips and mouth, as well as on her nasal mucosa. When she returned from Brazil the previous year, she had noted multiple skin lesions on her arm, which had since disappeared. Lymphadenopathy was noted on physical examination. A biopsy specimen was taken from the edge of an ulcer.

A section stained with hematoxylin and eosin showed macrophages containing small, oval parasites, measuring 2 to 3 μm (Fig. 26.1).

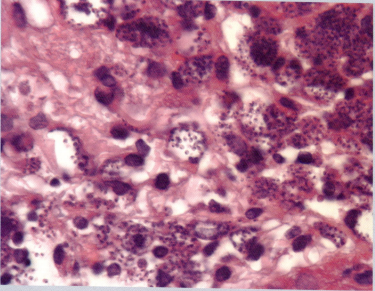

Figure 26.1

QUESTIONS

1. Which infection does this patient have? What is the name of the hemoflagellate causing her infection?

2. Name the four main species belonging to this complex.

3. Which vector is responsible for the transmission of this infection?

4. How does the life cycle of this parasite differ from that of other species?

5. How is the diagnosis of this infection made?

6. Do you think there is a connection between the patient's previous skin lesions on her arm and the mucosal lesions she now has? What course does this infection take if untreated?

7. Where is this hemoflagellate usually found? Where is the risk of exposure to infection greatest?

8. How is this infection treated?

ANSWERS

1. The patient has mucocutaneous leishmaniasis. In Brazil, the infection is known as espundia. The hemoflagellate causing her illness is a member of the *Leishmania braziliensis* complex. Members of this complex are considered to be a separate subgenus, *Viannia*, in contrast to all other *Leishmania* species, which belong to the subgenus *Leishmania*.

2. The four main species belonging to the *L. braziliensis* complex include *L. (V.) braziliensis, L. (V.) guyanensis, L. (V.) panamensis,* and *L. (V.) peruviana.*

3. Sand flies in the genera *Lutzomyia* and *Psychodopygus* act as the vectors for hemoflagellates in the *L. braziliensis* complex.

4. Members of the *L. braziliensis* complex develop in the hindgut of the sand fly vector, unlike the other species, which multiply in the midgut.

5. In areas where *Leishmania* is endemic, the diagnosis of mucocutaneous leishmaniasis is often based on clinical symptoms. The amastigotes may be detected in macrophages in Giemsa-stained smears of tissue specimens, or the promastigotes may be grown in culture. Specimens should be collected from the advancing margin of the lesion.

Animal inoculation methods may also be useful, although these methods are not commonly employed. PCR methods are quite sensitive and specific in diagnosing leishmaniasis. Although not performed in most clinical laboratories, these assays may be useful to screen patients in areas of endemic infection. The Montenegro skin test is useful for epidemiological purposes in screening large populations in areas of endemic infection. Serological methods are not very useful for the diagnosis of mucocutaneous leishmaniasis.

6. Large, multiple cutaneous lesions are common in infections with *L. braziliensis.* Mucosal lesions usually develop by metastasis from the original skin lesions located elsewhere on the body. The cutaneous lesions may be completely healed when mucosal ulcerations are present, or the two types of lesions may be present at the same time.

Without effective treatment, mucocutaneous leishmaniasis eventually progresses to involve the entire nasal mucosa, as well as the mucosa of the hard and soft palates, with extensive disfigurement. The nasal septum is involved, but no bone involvement occurs. Ulceration may extend to and destroy all the soft tissue of the nose, the lips, and soft palate. Secondary infection or the development of aspiration pneumonia may result in death.

7. *L. braziliensis* is found mostly in Latin America in the countries of Brazil (hence the name), Costa Rica, Ecuador, Nicaragua, Guatemala, Columbia, Venezuela, Peru, Paraguay, and Bolivia. The rain forest areas of these countries provide a habitat for the sand fly vectors, and a variety of forest animals serve as reservoirs. Timber cutters and other agriculture workers are at greatest risk of infection.

8. Lesions may be treated with pentavalent antimonials, such as antimony sodium gluconate (sodium stibogluconate), which is the drug of choice for the treatment of most cases of cutaneous leishmaniasis. However, the length of treatment is extended for mucocutaneous infection. Intravenous amphotericin B and intramuscular cycloguanil pamoate have also been reported to be effective.

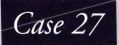

Case 27   A male immigrant from Mexico was seen in the dermatology clinic at a California hospital for examination of a large, painless, cutaneous ulcer on his ear. There was evidence of cartilage destruction in the area. A biopsy specimen was taken from the skin lesion and was sent to the laboratory for examination. A section stained with hematoxylin and eosin showed small, oval, nonflagellated protozoan amastigotes. A diagnosis of a blood-borne parasitic infection was made, based on the morphological appearance of the Giemsa-stained smear.

QUESTIONS

1. Which infection does this patient have? What is the name of the hemoflagellate causing his infection?

2. Name the three main species belonging to this complex.

3. Which vector is responsible for the transmission of this infection?

4. Describe the life cycle of this parasite.

5. What are the reservoirs for these parasites? Which populations are at particular risk of infection with these parasites?

6. How is the diagnosis of this infection made?

7. How is this infection treated?

ANSWERS

1. The patient has New World cutaneous leishmaniasis. A common name for this patient's lesion is chiclero ulcer or bay sore in Mexico. The hemoflagellate causing his illness is a member of the *Leishmania mexicana* complex.

2. The three main species belonging to the *L. mexicana* complex include *L. mexicana*, *L. amazonensis*, and *L. venezuelensis*. This complex belongs to the subgenus *Leishmania*, unlike the *L. braziliensis* complex, which belongs to the subgenus *Viannia*.

3. The *Lutzomyia* sand fly is the principal vector for hemoflagellates in the *L. mexicana* complex.

4. This parasite exists in two forms, the amastigote, which is a small, nonmotile, intracellular form, and the promastigote, which is an elongated, motile, extracellular form. The female sand fly vector infects a human by injecting the promastigote stage of the leishmania parasite into the skin while taking a blood meal. Promastigotes are phagocytized by macrophages. Intracellularly, the promastigotes transform into amastigotes. Amastigotes multiply in cells of various tissues, including macrophages, depending on the species. In cutaneous leishmaniasis, infected macrophages are confined to the skin. When a sand fly takes another blood meal, macrophages infected with amastigotes are ingested. Amastigotes transform into promastigotes in the midgut of the sand fly. Promastigotes multiply by longitudinal fission. They migrate to the proboscis of the sand fly, ready to be injected into another human, repeating the cycle.

5. Forest rodents act as reservoirs of infection for *L. mexicana*. Chicleros (so named because they collect chewing gum latex from chicle trees in the forests of Mexico), timber cutters, and other agriculture workers are at risk of infection with this parasite.

6. In areas where *Leishmania* is endemic, the diagnosis of cutaneous leishmaniasis is often made based on the clinical characteristics of the lesions. Although the growth of promastigotes in culture has been reported to be the most sensitive method for the diagnosis of cutaneous leishmaniasis, this procedure is costly and time-consuming and requires special equipment.

The amastigotes may be detected microscopically in macrophages in Giemsa-stained scrapings of lesions. Although the traditional recommendation is to collect specimens from the advancing indurated margin of the ulcer, a recent study suggests that collection of samples from the central region of the bottom of the lesion allows the detection of amastigotes with greater sensitivity. This study provided evidence that the use of a combination of bottom dermal scraping-extracted and margin dermal scraping-extracted specimens significantly enhancers the sensitivity of the microscopic examination.

Animal inoculation methods may also be useful, although these methods are not common. PCR amplification methods are quite sensitive and specific in the diagnosis of cutaneous leishmaniasis. Although not performed in most clinical laboratories due to their relatively high cost in developing countries and to the prerequisite for a specialized laboratory infrastructure, these assays may be useful for screening in areas of endemic infection. The Montenegro skin test is useful for epidemiological purposes in screening large populations in areas of endemic infection. A diameter of 5 mm or larger is considered positive. Serological methods are not very useful for the diagnosis of cutaneous leishmaniasis.

7. Systemic chemotherapy is recommended for the treatment of New World cutaneous leishmaniasis. Lesions may be treated with pentavalent antimonials, such as antimony sodium gluconate (sodium stibogluconate), which is the drug of choice for the treatment of cutaneous leishmaniasis. An exception is the Ethiopian form of diffuse infection, which is reported to respond better to pentamidine.

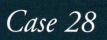

Case 28

A 23-year-old Peace Corps worker visited her family doctor complaining of flu-like symptoms, as well as persistent night sweats, headache, intermittent fever, and chills, which occurred at approximately 72-h intervals. She had recently returned from a 1-year tour of duty in Nicaragua. Hematological laboratory work was ordered.

The patient was slightly anemic with a hemoglobin level of 10.0 g/dl. Giemsa-stained thick and thin blood smears revealed very few infected red blood cells, which were of normal size. A rare schizont containing merozoites in a rosette pattern was seen. Band-like structures were seen intracellularly. Schüffner's dots were absent A characteristic trophozoite is shown in Fig. 28.1.

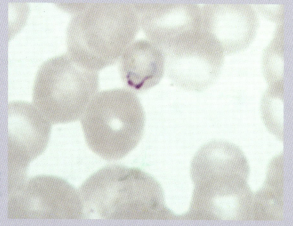

Figure 28.1

QUESTIONS

1. Which infection does this patient have? Which parasite is infecting her?

2. Describe the typical appearance of this parasite in thick and thin Giemsa-stained smears. What is the significance of the intracellular band-like structures?

3. Describe the clinical illness caused by this parasite. Do relapses or recrudescences occur? Compare these two terms.

4. Which serious complication may occur in this infection? Describe this syndrome.

5. What causes the chills and fever which are characteristic symptoms of this infection?

6. When should blood be collected when this infection is suspected?

7. How would this patient be treated?

ANSWERS

1. The patient has malaria caused by *Plasmodium malariae*.

2. Since *P. malariae* tends to infect older cells, parasitized erythrocytes are not enlarged. There are a limited number of infected cells. No eosinophilic stippling (Schüffner's dots) is observed. Older trophozoites may form band-like structures intracellularly, stretching across the red blood cell. Gametocytes of *P. malariae* may be difficult to distinguish from growing trophozoites but are ovoid when mature and slightly larger than mature trophozoites.

Early-ring-stage forms of the four species of *Plasmodium* are morphologically similar. However, the ring forms of *P. malariae* tend to be somewhat thicker than the others. The ring form of *Plasmodium* species consists of a light blue cytoplasm and a pink to red nucleus. Mature schizonts contain 6 to 12 merozoites, with an average of 8, in rosettes or irregular clusters. Brown-green pigment may be seen in the center of the mature schizont.

3. *P. malariae* causes quartan malaria, which is characterized by cycles and paroxysms every 72 h. Relapses may occur with *P. vivax* or *P. ovale* infections. This happens when resting-stage hypnozoites undergo secondary schizogony in the liver. A recrudescence refers to an increase in the number of intracellular parasites, when the malarial infection is not completely eradicated. Although relapses do not occur with *P. malariae* malaria, long-term recrudescences have been reported.

4. A complication of this type of malaria is the nephrotic syndrome. This syndrome is due to acute glomerulonephritis, which results when circulating antigen-antibody complexes are deposited in the glomeruli of the kidneys. Massive edema may occur in children with the nephrotic syndrome. Unlike most forms of the nephrotic syndrome, this complication associated with *P. malariae* infection is not treatable with steroids.

5. The characteristic paroxysms of malaria are due to the massive amounts of metabolic by-products released on rupture of the erythrocytes, with the release of large numbers of merozoites, following the schizogonic cycle in the human. The paroxysm may also be due to an allergic response of the patient to parasite antigens released from the erythrocytes.

6. Although the best way to make a species identification in the diagnosis of malaria is to examine blood smears prepared from blood drawn about halfway between chills, blood should be collected immediately when malaria is suspected. Since single smears may not reveal the malarial parasites, blood smears should be prepared every 6 to 8 h for up to 3 days to rule out this infection.

7. Therapy for malaria has become increasingly complex. A variety of drugs are available, and their use is based on their effects on the parasite at various stages of the life cycle. Although resistance of *P. falciparum* to chloroquine is well known, this drug is generally effective in treating infections with *P. vivax*, *P. malariae*, and *P. ovale*.

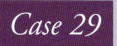

Case 29

A 45-year-old man who had been feeling unwell for several months visited his internist complaining of headache, dizziness, nausea, vomiting, extreme tiredness, and fever. The patient had been taking prednisone for a relapse of chronic ulcerative colitis.

On examination, the physician noted that the patient had nuchal rigidity and appeared confused. He performed a lumbar puncture. CSF was sent to the laboratory for bacterial and viral cultures. The Gram stain showed many neutrophils but no bacteria. To rule out amebic encephalitis, the physician asked that a wet mount be prepared from the patient's CSF. Microscopic examination of this preparation revealed motile amebic trophozoites. Cultures were negative for bacteria and viruses. A biopsy specimen containing the parasite causing this patient's infection is shown in Fig. 29.1.

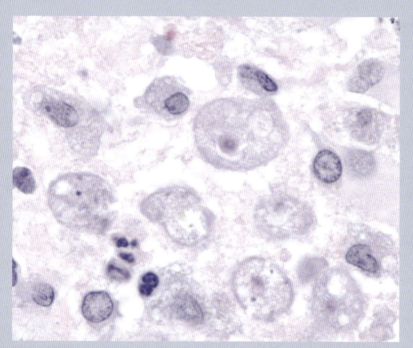

Figure 29.1

QUESTIONS

1. Which ameba would you expect to be causing this patient's infection? What is the name of this infection?

2. Which ameba may cause a more serious and acute CNS infection and may be confused with this parasite?

3. How can you distinguish between these amebae?

4. How do the infections caused by these two parasites differ?

5. How is the laboratory diagnosis of this infection made?

6. Does the ameba causing CNS infection in this patient cause other types of infections?

7. Which other free-living ameba, recently placed in the same genus as this parasite, causes a CNS infection in humans?

8. Why is there no satisfactory treatment available to treat this infection?

ANSWERS

1. This patient has GAE caused by an *Acanthamoeba* species, an opportunistic, free-living ameba.

2. *Naegleria fowleri* is a free-living ameba which causes PAM, a fulminant, rapidly progressive, and often fatal illness.

3. Although the ameboid stages of *Acanthamoeba* spp. and *N. fowleri* are similar in appearance, *Acanthamoeba* spp. have no flagellate stage. In *Acanthamoeba* infections, both trophozoites and cysts are found in brain tissue, while in *N. fowleri* infections, only trophozoites are found. Trophozoites of *Acanthamoeba* spp. characteristically have spiky projections (acanthopodia) on their pseudopods, unlike the blunt pseudopods of *N. fowleri*. Cysts are usually round with a single nucleus and a large karyosome. A double wall may be visible, with the outer wall being slightly wrinkled.

4. Infections with *Acanthamoeba* spp. are usually insidious, chronic, and prolonged, resulting in the formation of granulomas, due to the relatively slow process of tissue invasion, while *N. fowleri* usually causes a more fulminant and often rapidly progressive fatal infection. GAE occurs mostly in debilitated or chronically ill individuals or in immunocompromised patients, such as this patient, who was receiving steroids (prednisone) for his ulcerative colitis. The infection is unrelated to swimming. PAM generally occurs in healthy children and young adults, and is usually associated with swimming in contaminated water.

Unlike PAM, CNS invasion is secondary to infection elsewhere in the body in GAE. Since it is thought that the sinuses and lungs are the source of infection in immunocompromised patients with AIDS, it is likely that one of these sources is the primary site of infection for this patient. Amebae pass from the lower respiratory tract, or skin or mucosal ulcers, into the bloodstream and then to the brain. A granulomatous reaction occurs in the tissues of the CNS, as well as at the infected primary site.

5. The laboratory diagnosis of GAE is made by observing motile trophozoites of *Acanthamoeba* spp. in CSF or by the identification of *Acanthamoeba* cysts and trophozoites in brain tissue. The parasite may also be recovered from the infected primary tissues.

Although it is not easy to culture this parasite in vitro from CSF, improved medium formulations have been developed and have increased the success rate in the recovery of this parasite from clinical specimens. The amebae may be cultured by seeding agar plates with *Escherichia coli* bacterial cells, which serve as nutrients, before inoculating the medium with the patient's CSF. The agar plates are incubated at 37°C and examined daily for the telltale tracks, which may be seen in areas of bacterial growth. Plates should also be examined under low (10×) power daily for 10 days for amebic cysts and trophozoites, which can be scattered throughout the culture medium surface without obvious track lines.

6. This ameba is also known to cause a serious and painful eye infection, known as *Acanthamoeba* keratitis, in healthy people (see case 20). The greatest risk factor for developing *Acanthamoeba* keratitis is the use of homemade or commercial solutions that have been contaminated during use, or the use of an outdated product, as a cleansing agent for contact lenses.

7. *Balamuthia mandrillaris*, now known to cause GAE, an infection similar to that caused by *Acanthamoeba* spp., has recently joined *Acanthamoeba* in the family Acanthamoebidae.

8. There is no satisfactory treatment available to treat this infection because most cases of GAE have been diagnosed after death and there has been little opportunity to evaluate various therapeutic regimens.

REFERENCES

Carter, R., and K. N. Mendis. 2002. Evolutionary and historical aspects of the burden of malaria. *Clin. Microbiol. Rev.* **15**:564–594.

Centers for Disease Control and Prevention. 2003. Primary amebic meningoencephalitis—Georgia 2002. *Morb. Mortal. Wkly. Rep.* **52**:962–964.

Cox, F. E. G. 2002. History of human parasitology. *Clin. Microbiol. Rev.* **15**:595–612.

Garcia, L. S. 2001. *Diagnostic Medical Parasitology*, 4th ed. ASM Press, Washington, D.C.

Giraldo, M., R. W. D. Portela, M. Snege, P. G. Leser, M. E. Camargo, J. R. Mineo, and R. T. Gazzinelli. 2002. Immunoglobulin M (IgM)-glycoinositolphospholipid enzyme-linked immunosorbent assay: an immunoenzymatic assay for discrimination between patients with acute toxoplasmosis and those with persistent parasite-specific IgM antibodies. *J. Clin. Microbiol.* **40**:1400–1405.

Gray, J., L. V. von Stedingk, M. Gurtelschmid, and M. Granstrom. 2002. Transmission studies of *Babesia microti* in *Ixodes ricinus* ticks and gerbils. *J. Clin. Microbiol.* **40**:1249–1263.

Hay, S. I., M. Simba, M. Busolo, A. M. Noor, H. L. Guyatt, S. A. Ochola, and R. W. Snow. 2002. Defining and detecting malaria epidemics in the highlands of Western Kenya. *Emerg. Infect. Dis.* **8**:555–562.

Heelan, J. S., and F. W. Ingersoll. 2002. *Essentials of Human Parasitology.* Thomson Delmar Learning, Albany, N.Y.

Jelinek, T., Z. Bisoffi, L. Bonazzi, P. van Thiel, U. Bronner, A. de Frey, S. G. Gundersen, P. McWhinney, and D. Ripamonti. 2002. Cluster of African trypanosomiasis in travelers to Tanzanian national parks. *Emerg. Infect. Dis.* **8**:634–635.

Marciano-Cabral, F., and G. Cabral. 2003. *Acanthamoeba* spp. as agents of disease in humans. *Clin. Microbiol. Rev.* **16**:273–307.

Markell, E. K., D. T. John, and W. A. Krotoski. 1999. *Markell and Voge's Medical Parasitology*, 8th ed. The W. B. Saunders Co., Philadelphia, Pa.

Namdari, H., S. E. Pascucci, and E. J. Bottone. 2000. Well water as a source for *Acanthamoeba* keratitis. *Clin. Microbiol. Newsl.* **22**:53–55.

National Committee for Clinical Laboratory Standards. 2000. *Laboratory Diagnosis of Blood-borne Parasitic Diseases.* Approved guideline M15-A. National Committee for Clinical Laboratory Standards, Villanova, Pa.

Newman, R. D., A. M. Barber, J. Roberts, T. Holtz, R. W. Steketee, and M. E. Parise. 2002. Malaria surveillance—United States, 1999. *Morb. Mortal. Wkly. Rep.* **51**(SS-1):15–28.

Ramirez, J. R., S. Agudelo, C. Muskus, J. F. Alzate, C. Berberich, D. Barker, and I. D. Velez. 2000. Diagnosis of cutaneous leishmaniasis in Colombia: the sampling site within lesions influences the sensitivity of parasitological diagnosis. *J. Clin. Microbiol.* **38**:3768–3773.

Saran, R., M. C. Sharma, A. K. Gupta, S. P. Sinhar, and S. K. Kar. 1998. Diurnal periodicity of *Leishmania* amastigotes in peripheral blood of Indian kala-azar patients. *Acta Trop.* **68**:357–360.

Schuster, F. L. 2002. Cultivation of pathogenic and opportunistic free-living amebas. *Clin. Microbiol. Rev.* **15**:329–341.

Schuster, F. L., T. H. Dunnebacke, G. C. Booton, S. Yagi, C. K. Kohlmeier, C. Glaser, D. Vugia, A. Bakardjiev, P. Azimi, M. Maddux-Gonzalez, A. J. Martinez, and G. S. Visvesvara. 2003. Environmental isolation of *Balamuthia mandrillaris* associated with a case of amebic encephalitis. *J. Clin. Microbiol.* **41**:3175–3180.

Shenoy, S., G. Wilson, H. V. Prashanth, K. Vidyalakshmi, B. Dhanashree, and R. Bharath. 2002. Primary meningoencephalitis by *Naegleri fowleri*: first reported case from Mangalore, South India. *J. Clin. Microbiol.* 40:309–310.

Wever, P. C., Y. M. C. Henskins, P. A. Kager, J. Dankert, and T. van Gool. 2002. Detection of imported malaria with the Cell-DYN4000 hematology analyzer. *J. Clin. Microbiol.* 40: 4729–4731.

Zeibig, E. A. 1997. *Clinical Parasitology.* The W. B. Saunders Co., Philadelphia, Pa.

This section includes cases of infection with the helminths (worms) known as cestodes (tapeworms), trematodes (flukes), and intestinal nematodes (roundworms). These infections are usually diagnosed by finding eggs, larvae, or adult worms in fecal specimens. Helminth eggs are usually characteristic for that particular worm. The eggs are much larger than protozoan trophozoites and cysts and so are more readily visible microscopically. Characteristic features of helminth eggs include size and shape; the color and thickness of the eggshell are also important. Embryos are sometimes visible in the eggs.

Humans may be infected with the larval or adult form of cestodes, flatworms found in the phylum Platyhelminthes. Tapeworm infection may be diagnosed by microscopic detection of the eggs of these parasites during a traditional examination of feces for ova and parasites. Gravid proglottids of the tapeworm may also be present. Tapeworm larvae are not found in fecal specimens.

Taenia saginata and *Taenia solium* are known as the beef tapeworm and the pork tapeworm, respectively. In addition to causing intestinal infection, *T. solium* may cause cysticercosis. *Hymenolepis nana* is known as the dwarf tapeworm because it is the smallest tapeworm that infects humans; it requires no intermediate host.

Diphyllobothrium latum is the broad (or fish) tapeworm and is associated with fish consumption. *Dipylidium caninum*, the dog tapeworm, causes more infections in children, probably due to the close association of children with their pets. Hydatid cyst disease is caused by the cestode *Echinococcus granulosus*.

Trematodes (flukes) are also flatworms in the phylum Platyhelminthes. Fluke infections are also diagnosed by detection of the eggs of these parasites, although larvae and adult flukes are occasionally seen. Trematodes infecting humans include the sheep liver fluke, *Fasciola hepatica*, and the giant intestinal fluke, *Fasciolopsis buski*. The blood flukes, which live in blood vessels, are known as schistosomes; they include *Schistosoma mansoni*, *Schistosoma haematobium*, and *Schistosoma japonicum*. The eggs of these flukes may be distinguished by their morphological characteristics. The lung fluke *Paragonimus westermani*, along with nematodes that migrate through the lungs as part of their life cycles, may cause pulmonary symptoms. Eggs of this parasite may be found in sputum, as well as feces. *Clonorchis sinensis* is the Chinese liver fluke; infections with this species are common in the Far East.

Nematodes are roundworms in the phylum Aschelminthes. These are the most common intestinal helminths found in human infections. Most nematode infections are diagnosed by the detection of eggs or larvae in fecal specimens; adults are not usually found. The size and shape of the egg are constant for each species. The shape may be round or oval. For the detection of pinworm infection, the "Scotch tape test" is recommended over the traditional examination of fecal specimens for ova and parasites.

The appearance of the eggs of the intestinal nematode *Ascaris lumbricoides* varies in the fertilized and unfertilized states. Transmission of nematode infections may occur via the fecal-oral route by ingestion of eggs in food or water (for *Enterobius vermicularis, Ascaris lumbricoides,* and *Trichuris trichiura*) or by penetration of the skin by larval forms (for hookworms and *Strongyloides stercoralis*).

In addition to microbiological tests, other laboratory tests, including assays for liver enzyme levels, urinalysis, and hematology tests (including an eosinophil count), may aid in the diagnosis of infections with intestinal helminths. Radiology studies, such as computed tomography scans, might be helpful in the diagnosis of some of the cases described in this section.

Most patients infected with cestodes, trematodes, and intestinal nematodes present with gastrointestinal symptoms, especially diarrhea and abdominal pain. As with intestinal protozoan infections, travel history and place of residence are very important, as are the patient's dietary habits. The age of the patient is significant as well. Pinworm infection is more common in children.

Cultural habits play a role in the transmission of helminthic infections. Practices such as eating raw fish and vegetation (in some countries) predispose to infections with some of these parasites. Prevention of infection requires adherence to good personal hygiene practices and avoidance of contaminated food or water. The use of human waste (night soil) as fertilizer should be discouraged.

A variety of procedures, including surgery and the administration of drugs, are available to treat patients infected with cestodes, trematodes, or intestinal nematodes.

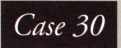

Case 30

An 8-year-old boy was not sleeping well, had been irritable, and had complained to his mother about anal itching and irritation. The boy's younger sibling also began to complain of similar symptoms. The children were taken to their pediatrician for evaluation. She ordered a parasitology laboratory test to provide a diagnosis. A worm egg seen microscopically enabled the laboratory to identify the worm causing the symptoms.

QUESTIONS

1. Which type of laboratory procedure would the physician have ordered to make a diagnosis? Which helminth is causing the children's discomfort? *Enterobius Vermicularis* *Transparent adhesive tape around the anal area. (Scotch tape test)*

2. How is this procedure performed?

3. How is the diagnosis made, using this procedure?

4. Describe the life cycle of this helminth.

5. How is the infection transmitted? *ingestion of eggs c contaminated food, hands or H2O*

6. Which intestinal protozoan has been associated with this helminthic infection? Explain.

7. Should this patient be treated?

mebendazole & Albendazole

ANSWERS

1. The physician should have ordered a cellophane tape preparation ("Scotch tape test") to confirm the diagnosis of enterobiasis (pinworm infection). The intestinal parasitic worm causing this infection is a nematode (roundworm), *Enterobius vermicularis*.

2. The specimen should be obtained late at night or early in the morning, after female worm migration has occurred and before the child has had a bowel movement. It is collected by applying transparent (not opaque) cellophane tape to the perianal area. The tape is then pressed onto a clean glass microscope slide. The slide is examined microscopically for the presence of typical eggs. Four to six slides prepared from specimens collected consecutively should be examined to rule out infection. A commercially available device called a Swoop Tube provides a more convenient method of specimen collection for the examination for pinworms. The female adult worm is occasionally found in stool specimens (the male worm is usually too small to see). The routine examination for ova and parasites is not recommended for the diagnosis of pinworm infection.

3. The eggs of *E. vermicularis* should be visible under the microscope. These eggs are oval and flattened on one side and have thick, colorless shells. They are up to 60 μm long by up to 30 μm wide. Larvae may be visible within the embryonated eggs. Adult worms are sometimes seen. The female worm, larger than the male, is 7 to 13 mm long; adult males are smaller and usually go unnoticed.

4. The life cycle of *E. vermicularis* is direct and begins with the deposition of partially embryonated eggs, usually at night, when the gravid female migrates from the intestine of the infected individual and cements the eggs onto the perianal skin. Infective eggs are readily dispersed into the environment. The female worm produces large numbers of eggs, which develop to the infectious stage within a few hours. The eggs may survive for several weeks at moderate temperature with high humidity. Once the embryonated egg is ingested, maturation to the adult stage occurs in the intestine after about 1 month.

5. Enterobiasis is a common parasitic infection, particularly in children, and is transmitted directly by the fecal-oral route or by ingestion or inhalation of embryonated ova. Eggs may be spread from contaminated fingers or fomites, such as bed linen, toilet seats, or clothing. Infection is found worldwide but is especially common in temperate climates. It is frequently spread among family members.

6. It is thought that the intestinal flagellate *Dientamoeba fragilis* may be transmitted in the ova of certain helminths, including *E. vermicularis* and *Ascaris lumbricoides*. This hypothesis, not yet proven, is based on the frequency of finding *D. fragilis* in patients infected with these helminths, as well as the detection by electron microscopy of structures resembling pinworm eggs containing *D. fragilis*. Simultaneous infections with both *D. fragilis* and *E. vermicularis* have frequently been reported.

7. Although asymptomatic patients are rarely treated, this patient showed symptoms and could be treated with pyrantel pamoate or mebendazole. Repeat treatment after 2 weeks is recommended to prevent reinfection by the ingestion of eggs remaining on bedclothes or on fomites after the first treatment. It is sometimes prudent to empirically treat an entire family to prevent recurrence of infection.

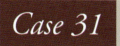

Case 31

A 32-year-old businessman from Europe arrived at an American emergency room suffering from diarrhea, indigestion, and abdominal pain in the right upper quadrant. He had a slightly enlarged liver. When questioned regarding his eating habits, the patient admitted to having a fondness for uncooked watercress. An order was written for a stool culture and examination for ova and parasites. Blood was collected for a cell count and liver function tests.

No enteric pathogenic bacteria were isolated from culture. Hematology results showed evidence of eosinophilia, with 15% eosinophils. The patient's liver enzyme levels were slightly elevated. The diagnosis was made microscopically after the observation of large, broad, ellipsoidal, brownish yellow operculated helminth eggs in the concentrated fecal specimen. A characteristic egg is shown in Fig. 31.1.

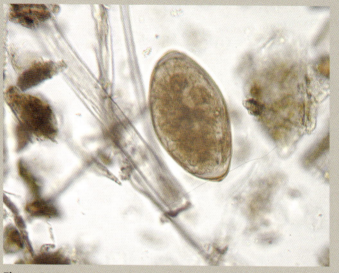

Figure 31.1

QUESTIONS

1. Which helminth might be causing this patient's infection?

2. Which other helminth produces eggs indistinguishable from the eggs described in this specimen?

3. Where is this parasite found geographically, and what are the usual symptoms of disease in humans?

4. How is the diagnosis of this infection usually made?

5. How does transmission of this helminth occur?

6. Describe the life cycle of this parasite.

7. Which other type of infection with this helminth may occur in areas of endemic infection?

8. How is this infection treated?

ANSWERS

1. The helminth causing this patient's infection is the sheep liver fluke, *Fasciola hepatica*.

2. The giant intestinal fluke, *Fasciolopsis buski*, produces large, operculated ova indistinguishable from those of *Fasciola hepatica*. However, the eggs of the latter parasite may be characterized by having a thickening at the abopercular end.

3. Although especially prevalent in South America, *F. hepatica* is found worldwide. Infection is especially common in areas where there is a close association of herbivores and humans. Symptoms of infection with the sheep liver fluke include abdominal pain, diarrhea, and indigestion. The liver may be damaged when the worm migrates through that organ. This depends on the worm burden. Mechanical irritation of the bile ducts is common. Obstruction of the biliary tract may occur.

4. A routine examination for ova and parasites should reveal the characteristic ova of *F. hepatica*, although multiple stool specimens may be required if the worm burden is low. The zinc sulfate flotation method is unsatisfactory for diagnosis, since the operculated ova do not float. The sedimentation concentration method is preferred. The low-power (10×) objective is usually adequate to identify *F. hepatica*, due to the large size of the ova.

5. The infection is transmitted by ingestion of raw water vegetation, such as watercress, bearing encysted metacercariae of *F. hepatica*, as a result of growing in water contaminated by herbivores. Infection may also be transmitted by ingestion of contaminated water containing free-floating metacercariae.

6. Unembryonated eggs are passed in the feces of infected animals. The miracidium develops, escapes from the egg, and infects the snail, which acts as the first intermediate host. Cercariae develop in the snail and are released into the water, where they encyst, forming metacercariae on vegetation. Human infection follows ingestion of uncooked contaminated vegetation. Metacercariae may also become detached from vegetation, thus contaminating the water. The metacercariae excyst in the duodenum. Larvae pass through the wall of the intestine and migrate into the liver and bile ducts. The adult worms of this helminth reside in the large bile ducts and gallbladder in humans, rather than in the intestine. Eggs are carried by the bile fluid into the intestine and are passed in the feces.

7. In areas of endemic infection, such as the Middle East, where uncooked sheep and goat livers are eaten, adult worms or larvae may attach to the pharyngeal mucosa, causing a condition known as the halzoun syndrome. Edema and congestion of the soft palate may occur, with resulting pain, dyspnea, dysphagia, and, occasionally, suffocation. Although, halzoun was originally thought to be an uncommon condition resulting from infection with *F. hepatica*, recent reports suggest that most, if not all, cases of halzoun are caused by nymphs of pentastomes (linguatulids), which are wormlike parasites inhabiting the respiratory passages of carnivorous reptiles, birds, and mammals.

8. Patients infected with *F. hepatica* may be treated with several drugs, including praziquantel, bithionol, and triclabendazole. Although not easily obtained, triclabendazole shows few side effects and may become the drug of choice in treating this infection.

Case 32

A 26-year-old male university student studying in Mexico City was in good health until he experienced a seizure at home in the United States during Christmas vacation. He had complained of headaches for several weeks, which he attributed to the stress caused by his final examinations, and had vomited several times. His parents brought him to the emergency room, where he was examined.

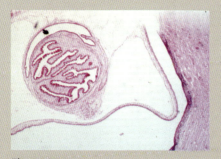

Figure 32.1

When his neurological examination showed no focal abnormalities, a computed tomogram was ordered. Several calcified lesions were observed in both cerebral hemispheres. A parasitic infection was suspected. A brain biopsy revealed the parasite causing the patient's symptoms (Fig. 32.1). Blood and cerebrospinal fluid specimens were submitted for laboratory analysis to confirm the diagnosis.

QUESTIONS

1. Which parasitic infection do you think this patient has? Which helminth causes this infection? _ T. Solium

2. How do you diagnose extraintestinal infection with this parasite?

3. How do humans acquire this infection? auto infection

4. Which other type of infection may be caused by this helminth?

5. How do you diagnose this type of infection with this parasite? ova in faeces

6. Which treatment is available for this infection?

albendazole & mcebendazole

ANSWERS

1. This patient has neurocysticercosis, which is caused by the pork tapeworm *Taenia solium*.

2. Cysticerci may develop in any tissue but are more likely to cause symptoms in the central nervous system. Neurocysticercosis is more serious than intestinal infection and is the most common helminthic disease of the central nervous system. This disease is also the most common cause of adult-onset epilepsy worldwide. It may be diagnosed by radiographic findings such as computed tomograms or magnetic resonance imaging studies. These studies usually show multiple intracranial lesions.

Surgical removal of intracranial cysts and demonstration of the tapeworm scolex bearing suckers and hooks is useful to confirm the diagnosis. Although serum and cerebrospinal fluid may be submitted for serological studies, these tests are frequently negative in patients with cysticercosis of the central nervous system.

3. The larval stage of *T. solium* is called a cysticercus or bladder worm. Proglottids of adult worms containing eggs are passed in human feces. When the eggs of this parasite are accidentally ingested by humans (instead of pigs, which usually act as intermediate hosts for this parasite), the human replaces the pig as an intermediate host, a larva develops, and a condition known as cysticercosis may arise.

The oncosphere develops and the outer eggshell disintegrates in the small intestine. The oncosphere escapes from the egg and invades the intestinal wall. It then may enter a blood vessel and invade the body tissues, especially tissues and organs of the nervous system, where it causes neurocysticercosis. In this infection, the larva does not mature into an adult tapeworm in the human.

4. Pigs become infected after ingesting embryonated eggs of *T. solium*. The eggs develop into infective larvae or cysticerci in the muscles of the pig. Humans may develop intestinal infection with *T. solium* by ingesting uncooked pork which contains the cysticercus larvae of the parasite. Stomach juices digest the larva out of the meat. The scolex of the larva attaches to the mucosa of the small intestine, and the adult tapeworm develops. Eggs are produced and are passed in human feces.

5. Intestinal infection with *T. solium* is diagnosed by recovery of characteristic eggs or gravid proglottids in human feces. Gravid proglottids are longer than wide and contain a branched uterus with a central uterine stem from which lateral branches extend. These proglottids may be differentiated from those of the beef tapeworm, *T. saginata*, by counting the number of uterine branches. *T. solium* has 7 to 13 branches, while *T. saginata* has 15 to 20. This procedure may be performed by India ink injection staining or in living preparations.

Eggs are usually not found in large numbers. The round, yellow-brown, thick-shelled eggs of *T. solium* and *T. saginata* have radially striated coats and often contain a recognizable oncosphere with six hooks, but the eggs of these tapeworms cannot be distinguished from each other. The scolex of *T. solium,* which is not usually found in feces, is characterized by having four suckers and a rostellum with hooklets. These hooks attach to the intestinal wall. The scolex is sometimes recovered by purgation.

6. Although surgical removal of the cysticerci is recommended when possible, medical intervention is available. Treatment with praziquantel and niclosamide is effective against this parasite.

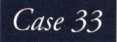

Case 33

A 19-year-old woman who had recently returned from a semester of schooling in Costa Rica had been suffering from crampy abdominal pain and diarrhea for just over a week. After a physical examination, which was unremarkable, her family physician ordered a stool culture and also gave the patient vials of preservatives (10% formalin and polyvinyl alcohol) to collect specimens for an examination for fecal parasites.

The stool culture was negative for enteric bacterial pathogens. Microscopic examination of a concentrated wet-mount preparation made from one of the 10% formalin vials revealed several types of nematode eggs. These eggs had thick shells and were oval, with some being more broadly oval than others. One type of egg is shown in Fig. 33.1. Several eggs lacked the mammillated outer covering found on the majority of eggs. This egg type is shown in Fig. 33.2.

A diagnosis of infection with an intestinal nematode was made on the basis of microscopic analysis.

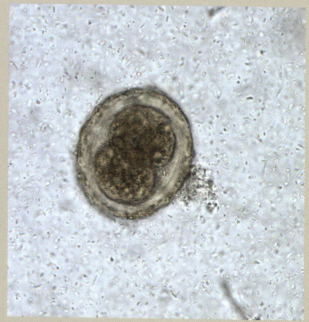

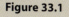
Figure 33.1

QUESTIONS

1. Which nematodes are most likely to cause human intestinal infection?

2. Which nematode would you suspect of causing this patient's infection? Explain the variable appearance of the nematode eggs seen microscopically.

3. Describe the life cycle of this helminth.

4. How is this infection transmitted?

5. Describe the clinical symptoms of this infection.

6. Which complications may cause this infection to be life-threatening?

7. How is this infection treated?

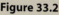
Figure 33.2

ANSWERS

1. The most common clinically significant nematodes which may cause human intestinal infection are the hookworms *Ancylostoma duodenale* and *Necator americanus*, the whipworm *Trichuris trichiura*, the pinworm *Enterobius vermicularis*, the threadworm *Strongyloides stercoralis*, and the giant intestinal roundworm *Ascaris lumbricoides*.

2. The patient is probably infected with the large roundworm, *Ascaris lumbricoides*. Both fertilized and unfertilized ova may be seen in the same stool specimen from patients infected with *A. lumbricoides*. Eggs passed in the feces are usually in the one-cell stage. The fertilized egg is broadly oval and measures up to 75 μm long and up to 50 μm wide. The egg usually has a thick, transparent shell, usually stained golden brown with bile, surrounded by a mammillated outer covering. Unfertilized eggs are more elongated (up to 90 μm long), have thinner walls, and show disorganized globular internal contents. Mammillations may be prominent and scattered irregularly or may be almost absent. When the mammillated outer covering is completely absent from fertile or infertile eggs, the egg is said to be decorticated.

Unfertilized eggs do not float if the zinc sulfate flotation concentration method is used, because they are too heavy. The ethyl acetate sedimentation concentration technique is preferred for their recovery.

3. Fertilized eggs, passed in human feces, become infective in warm, moist soil within 2 weeks. Humans become infected after ingesting food contaminated with infective eggs. After ingestion, embryonated eggs containing second-stage larvae pass into the small intestine, where they hatch. The larvae do not mature immediately but penetrate the intestinal wall and migrate via the hepatic portal circulation to the liver, the right side of the heart, the pulmonary vessels, and the lungs. They eventually reach the trachea and pharynx. The larvae are swallowed and pass into the small intestine, where they mature and where the male and female mate. About 2 months after infection, egg deposition occurs and the cycle begins again. In the absence of males, females produce infertile eggs.

4. Ascariasis occurs worldwide and is transmitted by the fecal-oral route. Humans become infected by the ingestion of embryonated eggs from soil contaminated with human waste. This infection is therefore common in many developing countries where human feces are used as fertilizer. Fertilized eggs are passed in the feces. Maturation occurs in the soil, with formation of the second-stage larvae within approximately 2 weeks.

Trichuris trichiura infection may occur simultaneously with *Ascaris* infection. This is probably because the eggs of both of these helminths require similar soil conditions for development and are more common in warm, moist areas of the world.

5. Patients with ascariasis usually present with diarrhea and abdominal pains. However, pulmonary symptoms may be evident during the pulmonary phase of larval migration. Signs of pneumonitis may occur if the larval burden is high. The bronchial epithelium may be damaged as the larvae migrate from the lung tissue into the alveoli. Tissue reactions may occur in the liver or lungs.

The presence of adult worms in the intestine usually causes few symptoms unless the worm burden is high. Nutritional deficiencies related to the worm burden may develop, particularly in children.

6. This large worm may be voided in the feces or may emerge from the anus. The tendency of adult ascarids to migrate, especially when fever occurs or during the use of general anesthesia, may lead to life-threatening situations. Migration may lead to obstruction such as intestinal blockage or, if the worm migrates out of the nose or mouth, asphyxia.

7. Mebendazole or albendazole may be used to treat ascariasis in both children and adults. Pyrantel pamoate is an alternative drug. Although effective in killing adult worms, the drugs may be ineffective in eliminating the migrating larvae. Intestinal obstruction may be treated by nasogastric suctioning until vomiting is controlled. Surgical intervention may be needed if certain body sites are involved. Worms have been removed from the biliary tract in order to prevent pancreatitis or cholangitis. Surgery might also be necessary if complete intestinal obstruction occurs.

Case 34

A 42-year-old man had traveled to Egypt on business 6 months before his presentation to the emergency department with complaints of painful urination and the presence of blood in his urine. During his stay in Egypt, his business partners treated him to a river tour, which included swimming in the local river. The emergency room physician ordered a urinalysis and a urine culture to rule out kidney abnormalities or a urinary tract infection.

Culture results were negative for bacteria. Urinalysis revealed normal glucose levels and proteinuria. Many red blood cells (hematuria) plus a few white blood cells were seen on microscopic examination of the urine sediment. Oval helminth eggs (shown in Fig. 34.1) bearing prominent, terminal spines were also present in moderate numbers.

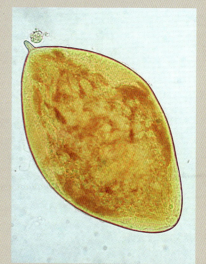

Figure 34.1

QUESTIONS

1. Which helminth is causing this patient's infection?

2. How is this infection transmitted?

3. Describe the appearance of the ova of this species of helminth. How do these ova compare with those of other members of this genus?

4. How is this infection diagnosed? Which types of specimens should be collected?

5. Describe the "hatching test" and how it is used in the diagnosis of this infection.

6. Describe the life cycle of this helminth.

7. What is the association of this infection with bladder cancer?

8. How is this infection treated?

ANSWERS

1. The helminth causing this patient's infection is the blood fluke, *Schistosoma haematobium*.

2. Unlike other trematode infections, which are acquired by ingestion of metacercariae, this infection is transmitted to humans when free-living cercariae, after their release from a snail, directly penetrate human skin. Cercariae contain glands that produce material which aids the penetration of the skin. Transmission usually occurs while humans are swimming or bathing in contaminated water

3. A schistosome egg lacks the operculum present in the eggs of other trematodes. Spines are characteristically found on schistosome eggs. The egg of *S. haematobium* is light yellow-brown, has an oblong shape and a single prominent terminal spine, and measures up to 170 by 70 μm. That of *S. mansoni* has a similar shape but is slightly larger, measuring up to 180 by 73 μm, and has a well-developed lateral spine. The smallest eggs, which are up to 100 μm long and up to 65 μm wide, are those of *S. japonicum;* these eggs are round, and the small lateral spines may not be visible.

4. Infection with *S. haematobium* is diagnosed by the detection of eggs in urine specimens, although eggs are sometimes found in fecal specimens as well as in semen. Eggs can be detected in the urine only after the worms mature, which may take as long as 3 months. Diagnosis may require examination of multiple urine specimens if the patient has a light worm burden. Peak egg excretion occurs between noon and 3 p.m. Urine specimens collected without preservatives during this time or over a 24-h period are recommended. Microscopic examination should be performed following centrifugation or sedimentation. The membrane filter technique using Nuclepore filters may be used to make a diagnosis of infection with *S. haematobium*. Travel history may also be helpful in the diagnosis of schistosomiasis.

5. Hatching tests may be used in the diagnosis of chronic schistosomiasis to determine egg viability when the worm burden is light. The test is designed to mimic conditions in nature, with spring water and sunlight. The unpreserved urine specimen is placed in water in a flask or beaker. The sides of the vessel are covered with aluminum foil to prevent light entry. A light source is used to project a perpendicular light beam through the water at the top. Miracidia will hatch from live eggs and concentrate in the light. The motile larvae, which swim around, may be seen with a hand lens and may also be viewed under a dissecting microscope. Observations should be made every 30 min for 4 h.

6. Free-swimming cercariae penetrate human skin. The schistosome cercariae lose their bifurcated tails following skin penetration. These forms enter the circulation, mature to adulthood in the portal blood, and reside in the blood vessels around the urinary bladder. After male and female worms mate, eggs are produced, are extruded from the adult worms residing in the venules of the urinary bladder, and work their way through the bladder wall. The eggs are excreted in the urine. They are fully embryonated when they leave the body. The miracidium is mature when it is released from the egg in water. It finds and penetrates a suitable snail host. Cercariae are produced and released from the snail into the water.

7. *S. haematobium* was classified by the International Agency for Research on Cancer as a carcinogenic agent in 1997. Chronic infection with this parasite has been associated with carcinoma of the urinary bladder. Squamous cell carcinoma of the bladder is probably associated with continuous exposure to *N*-nitroso compounds (carcinogens) produced as a result of secondary bacterial infections. This type of carcinoma is associated with high or moderate worm burdens; transitional cell carcinoma of the bladder occurs more frequently in geographic areas where patients have lighter worm burdens.

8. Praziquantel is the drug of choice to treat infections with *S. haematobium*, although it is ineffective against immature stages of schistosomes. A single oral dose is usually adequate for treatment; it has mild and transient side effects. An alternative drug is the organophosphorus cholinesterase inhibitor metrifonate. This drug is also given orally over several weeks and has minimal side effects.

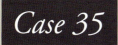

Case 35

A 45-year-old male professor visiting from Korea, who was lecturing in the United States, reported to an outpatient clinic suffering from abdominal pain, diarrhea, and fever. A stool specimen was submitted for culture, and three specimens were collected daily and sent to the laboratory for ova and parasite examinations. Blood was drawn for hematology studies.

The blood specimen sent to a laboratory revealed eosinophilia, with 18% eosinophils. The stool culture was negative for bacterial pathogens. The stool specimens submitted for parasitological examination were positive for helminth eggs. These were described as small, delicate-looking, flask-shaped eggs having brownish shells and with distinct "shoulders" around the operculum. A small comma-shaped knob was noted opposite the operculum. The egg is shown in Fig. 35.1.

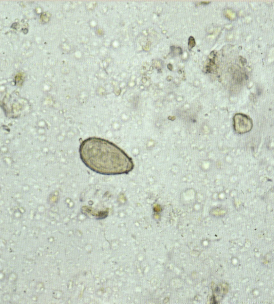

Figure 35.1

QUESTIONS

1. Which intestinal parasite is causing this patient's infection?

2. How is this helminth detected?

3. Which aspect of the patient's history correlates with his infection?

4. Describe the life cycle of this parasite.

5. How might this infection lead to obstructive jaundice?

6. How is this infection treated?

ANSWERS

1. The parasite causing this patient's infection is the Chinese liver fluke, *Clonorchis sinensis*.

2. The eggs of this trematode, sometimes observed in unconcentrated preparations from fresh fecal specimens or specimens preserved in 10% formalin vials, are oval with prominent shoulders surrounding the operculum. The brownish yellow eggs measure 15 by 30 μm and appear delicate. Due to their small size, it is recommended that the high dry (40×) objective be used to examine the wet mount. The zinc sulfate flotation method is unsatisfactory for diagnosis, since the operculated eggs do not float. The sedimentation concentration method is preferred. It may be necessary to examine multiple stool specimens to detect the eggs of *C. sinensis*. The eggs may also be recovered from duodenal aspirates.

3. This patient was a visiting professor from Korea. The Chinese liver fluke is common in the Far East, including Korea, Japan, Vietnam, and Taiwan. It is acquired from ingestion of infected uncooked or poorly cooked fish, which in these countries may be steamed or served as sushi.

4. After the embryonated egg of *C. sinensis* is ingested by a snail, it hatches and the miracidium infects the snail. After sporocyst and rediae generations are produced, cercariae are released and encyst as metacercariae in freshwater fish. Humans are infected by ingesting the metacercariae encysted in raw or undercooked fish.

Metacercariae excyst in the duodenum, enter the common bile duct, and travel into the bile capillaries. The adult worms mature and deposit eggs in the small bile capillaries. The fully embryonated eggs pass in bile fluid to the feces, where they leave the host. Dogs and cats serve as reservoirs of infection.

5. Heavy worm burdens with *C. sinensis* may result from repeated infections over several years. In these cases, bile ducts may become thickened, resulting in obstruction of the biliary tract, jaundice, and enlargement and functional impairment of the liver. Multiple liver abscesses may develop.

C. sinensis was classified by the International Agency for Research on Cancer in 1997 as a carcinogenic agent. In chronic infections, complications such as cholelithiasis and cholangiocarcinoma may lead to death. Acute pancreatitis has also occurred.

6. Praziquantel is the drug of choice to treat infections with *C. sinensis*. There are few side effects, although this drug should not be used during pregnancy. Albendazole is an alternative agent.

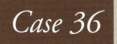

Case 36

A 64-year-old female American tourist had just returned from a Scandinavian vacation. Her history revealed that she had been particularly fond of eating the freshwater fish served in the Scandinavian restaurants. Soon after her return to the United States, she reported to an emergency room suffering from digestive disturbances including diarrhea and abdominal pain. A stool specimen was submitted for bacterial culture and microscopic examination for ova and parasites.

The bacterial culture was negative for enteric pathogens. The microscopic examination of a wet mount revealed large, oval, operculated helminth eggs. A typical helminth egg is shown in Fig. 36.1.

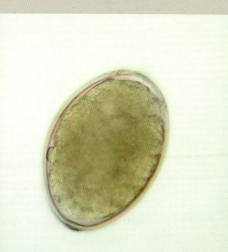

Figure 36.1

QUESTIONS

1. Which tapeworm is causing this patient's infection?

2. How does the genus name of this helminth reflect the appearance of the scolex?

3. How do the eggs of this helminth differ from those of other tapeworms? With which other helminth may this parasite be confused?

4. What is the association between the patient's history and her infection?

5. Describe the life cycle of this tapeworm. Why would you consider the life cycle to be complex?

6. Describe the appearance of the proglottids of this tapeworm.

7. Discuss the relationship between this helminth and pernicious anemia.

8. How is this infection treated?

ANSWERS

1. This patient is infected with the broad or fish tapeworm, *Diphyllobothrium latum*, which is found worldwide. Other species found in South America and Japan include *D. pacificum, D. dendriticum,* and *D. nihonkaiense.*

2. *D. latum* has a spoon-shaped scolex with two shallow, longitudinal sucking grooves, called bothria, one on the ventral surface and one on the dorsal surface. The scolex lacks the rostellum, suckers, and hooks found on most tapeworm scolices.

3. *D. latum* is the only tapeworm that produces operculated eggs. The operculated eggs of the lung fluke *Paragonimus westermani* may be confused with these eggs. However, the lung fluke eggs have opercular shoulders, unlike the tapeworm egg shown in Fig. 36.1. The tapeworm ovum may have a knob at the abopercular end.

4. The patient had recently returned from a Scandinavian vacation, where she had dined on freshwater fish. Diphyllobothriasis, although endemic in parts of the United States, is found in Scandinavia, Latin America, Asia, and Africa and is acquired by ingestion of tapeworm larvae in raw or undercooked freshwater fish such as salmon, perch, and trout.

5. The life cycle of *D. latum* (the broad or fish tapeworm) is complex because it involves two intermediate hosts and several larval stages. The adult tapeworm resides in the small intestine. After cross-fertilization occurs (the cestodes are hermaphroditic), eggs are produced and the unembryonated eggs are passed in human feces. Multiple attached proglottids are also often passed. After several weeks of development, a small ciliated embryo known as a coracidium is released. This embryo swims around and infects the first intermediate host, a crustacean known as a copepod, often in the genus *Cyclops.*

The second larval stage, known as a procercoid larva, develops in the copepod. The second intermediate host, a freshwater fish, ingests the copepod. The infective plerocercoid larva develops in the flesh of the fish. The fish containing the plerocercoid larvae may be eaten by a larger fish. This fish, in turn, may be eaten by a still larger fish, until the final fish intermediate host may contain many plerocercoid larvae. When the infected raw or undercooked fish is eaten by a suitable mammalian host, this results in infection. The scolex emerges and attaches to the intestinal wall. Maturation of the tapeworm occurs in the small intestine.

6. The proglottids of *D. latum*, often passed in chains, are much wider than long (hence the name "broad" tapeworm). The uterus is a coiled tube in the center of the proglottid. The arrangement of the uterus has been described as rosette shaped.

7. Diphyllobothriasis has been associated with a condition similar to pernicious anemia in a small number of individuals. A vitamin B_{12} deficiency may arise when this vitamin is absorbed by *D. latum* from the host intestinal tract.

8. Both praziquantel and niclosamide are recommended agents for treating infections with *D. latum.*

A 66-year-old farmer from the southeastern United States was seen for a routine annual physical examination. Aside from vague gastrointestinal complaints and fatigue, he had been well. The patient's physician ordered a stool culture for bacterial pathogens. Three specimens collected on alternate days were also submitted for examination for ova and parasites. No bacterial pathogens were identified, but a moderate number of helminth eggs were detected in two of the three fecal specimens. A typical egg is shown in Fig. 37.1.

A single nematode larva was also observed in one fecal specimen. This specimen had inadvertently sat overnight at room temperature before being processed. The larva is shown in Fig. 37.2.

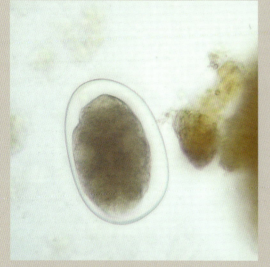

Figure 37.1

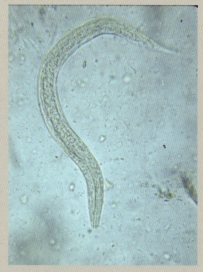

Figure 37.2

QUESTIONS

1. Based on the patient's symptoms and the morphology of the egg shown in Fig. 37.1, which two helminths are possible causes of the patient's symptoms?

2. Compare the geographical occurrence of these two helminths.

3. Would you expect to find both eggs and larvae of these helminths in an infected patient's stool specimen? Explain.

4. Describe the two larval stages of these helminths. Which other nematode has a larval form that may be confused with that shown in Fig. 37.2?

5. What causes the characteristic anemia that may occur in children heavily infected with this parasite?

6. How is this infection transmitted to humans?

7. Describe the life cycles of these helminths.

8. How is this infection treated?

ANSWERS

1. Based on the patient's symptoms and the morphological appearance of the helminth egg shown in Fig. 37.1, the hookworm *Necator americanus* is probably causing the infection. Although the eggs of this hookworm are indistinguishable from those of *Ancylostoma duodenale*, the latter hookworm is not found in the United States.

2. "New World" hookworm infection, caused by *N. americanus*, occurs predominantly in North and South America. It is the only hookworm found in these areas but is the native hookworm in southern Africa. "Old World" hookworm infection, caused by *A. duodenale*, is found mostly in Africa, India, China, southern Europe, and Japan. Both types of hookworm may be found in Brazil, India, China, Indonesia, and Southeast Asia. Today, since widespread international travel is commonplace, either parasite may be encountered worldwide, and geographical boundaries may disappear.

3. Although hookworm infections are usually diagnosed by the detection of characteristic eggs in human feces, the egg occasionally hatches in the feces, producing a rhabditiform larva, with the morphological appearance of the larva shown in Fig. 37.2. The larva was recovered from a specimen that had sat at room temperature overnight before being examined, which would account for the development of the larva.

4. It is necessary to distinguish the hookworm larva from the larvae of *Strongyloides stercoralis*, which requires different therapy and may cause a more severe type of infection. The hookworm rhabditiform larva (which is the noninfective free-living form) is characterized by a prominent buccal cavity and a small genital primordium. These characteristics help to distinguish the hookworm larva from the larva of *S. stercoralis*, whose rhabditiform larval form has a short buccal cavity and a prominent genital primordium. The hookworm filariform larva (the infective form) is not capable of living independently and must find a host. This form has an esophagus notably shorter than that of the filariform larva of *S. stercoralis* and a long, pointed tail.

5. In chronic hookworm infections in children, when a large number of worms are present, the loss of blood may result in iron deficiency anemia. Although the diet should provide enough iron to counteract the activity of the hookworms, inadequate nutrition in third-world countries may not prevent this condition.

6. Hookworm infection is acquired when the filariform larvae penetrate the skin, usually the hands or feet, from contaminated soil. It is most often acquired by individuals who walk barefoot in feces-contaminated soil.

7. The life cycles of *N. americanus* and *A. duodenale* are identical. The infection is initiated with the penetration of the skin by the filariform (third-stage) larvae from contaminated soil. The larvae enter the circulation, migrate to the lungs, trachea, and pharynx, and are swallowed. Maturation of the larval stage occurs in the intes-

tine, when the worms attach to the intestinal mucosa by means of their well-developed mouth parts. Eggs are produced in the intestine and are passed in the feces. The eggs hatch to produce rhabditiform larvae, which develop into third-stage (infective-stage) filariform larvae in the soil.

A minor means of hookworm transmission is ingestion of vegetables or dirt harboring filariform larvae. Ancylostomiasis has been transmitted through breast milk and possibly across the placenta.

8. Adequate nutrition may help to alleviate symptoms, but it does not cure the infection. Mebendazole, albendazole, or pyrantel pamoate may be used to treat hookworm disease, although low doses of pyrantel pamoate are not effective in eliminating infection with *A. duodenale*.

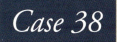

Case 38

A 36-year-old woman presented to her family practitioner complaining of diarrhea, mild indigestion, and slight abdominal pain. Blood was drawn for a complete blood count (CBC). The patient was instructed to submit a stool specimen for routine culture. Three stool specimens were collected for ova and parasite examination on alternate days, placed in vials of 10% formalin and poly-vinyl alcohol, and taken to the hospital laboratory for analysis.

The stool culture was reported negative for enteric bacterial pathogens. The blood count revealed an increase in the percentage of circulating eosinophils, which was 19%. On examination of the concentrated sediments for ova and parasites, several yellow-brown, spherical, thick-shelled helminth eggs measuring 30 to 40 μm in diameter were seen in each specimen. These eggs were characterized by radial striations. A typical egg is shown in Fig. 38.1. Six-hooked oncospheres were present in the eggs. Gravid tapeworm proglottids were also detected in the stool specimen; they contained 15 to 20 lateral uterine branches when stained with India ink.

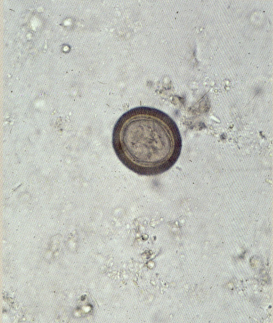

Figure 38.1

QUESTIONS

1. Which tapeworm is causing this patient's illness?

2. How is infection with this parasite acquired?

3. Name the two species of this genus which cause human disease. Can they be distinguished by the morphological appearance of their eggs?

4. Can these two tapeworms be distinguished by the appearance of their proglottids? Explain.

5. Compare the morphology of the scolex of these two tapeworms.

6. Why is it important to distinguish between these two tapeworms?

7. How is this infection treated?

ANSWERS

1. The tapeworm causing this patient's infection is the beef tapeworm *Taenia saginata*.

2. Human intestinal infection with *T. saginata* is acquired by ingestion of uncooked or insufficiently cooked beef containing the cysticercus larvae of the parasite.

3. The two species of *Taenia* which cause human infection are *T. solium*, the pork tapeworm and *T. saginata*, the beef tapeworm. The spherical, yellow-brown, thick-shelled eggs of *T. saginata* and *T. solium*, which both have radial striations and may be confused with pollen grains, are morphologically indistinguishable.

4. *T. saginata* and *T. solium* may be distinguished by microscopic examination of their gravid proglottids after India ink injection staining. Proglottids are longer than wide and contain a branched uterus with a central uterine stem. Lateral branches extend from this stem. The beef tapeworm proglottid measures approximately 17 by 19 mm and has 15 to 20 lateral uterine branches on each side of the uterus; the pork tapeworm proglottid measures 11 by 5 mm and has 7 to 13 lateral uterine branches.

5. The scolex of *T. solium* is characterized by having four suckers and a rostellum with hooklets. These hooks attach to the intestinal mucosa. The scolex of *T. saginata* also has four suckers but no rostellum or hooklets.

6. Although both *T. saginata* and *T. solium* cause intestinal tapeworm infection, only *T. solium* causes cysticercosis. This infection may occur if the eggs of the pork tapeworm are accidentally ingested by humans (instead of pigs). The human then acts as an intermediate host. The oncosphere develops, escapes from the egg, and invades the body tissues, especially tissues and organs of the nervous system, causing neurocysticercosis. Humans infected by eggs produce only cysticerci and not adult worms.

7. Praziquantel is an effective agent to treat taeniasis caused by *T. saginata*. Niclosamide is an acceptable alternate choice.

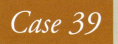

A 44-year-old man on a business trip to the United States from Asia presented to the emergency department with symptoms of diarrhea and abdominal pain. A stool specimen was sent to the laboratory for culture. Three stool specimens were collected on alternate days and sent for routine examinations for ova and parasites. Blood was drawn for a CBC.

The culture was negative for enteric pathogens. The patient was found to have eosinophilia. The wet mounts from the concentrated stool specimens revealed large, ellipsoidal, operculated helminth eggs with thin, transparent shells (Fig. 39.1). A diagnosis of a trematode (fluke) infection was made based on the appearance of the egg.

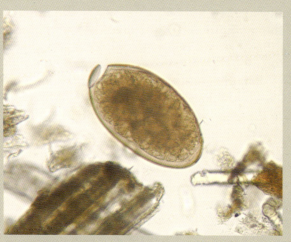

Figure 39.1

QUESTIONS

1. Which helminth might be causing this patient's infection?

2. Which other helminth produces eggs indistinguishable from the eggs described in this specimen?

3. Where is this parasite found geographically, and what are the usual symptoms of disease in humans?

4. Describe the life cycle of this parasite.

5. How can this infection be prevented?

6. How is this infection treated?

ANSWERS

1. The helminth causing this patient's infection is the giant intestinal fluke, *Fasciolopsis buski*. It is the largest fluke that inhabits humans.

2. The sheep liver fluke, *Fasciola hepatica*, produces large, operculated eggs indistinguishable from those of *Fasciolopsis buski*. Although the eggs of *Fasciola hepatica* may be characterized by having a thickening at the abopercular end, this characteristic does generally not allow differentiation between the two parasites. When specific identification is in doubt, eggs may be reported as belonging to the *Fasciolopsis buski*/*Fasciola hepatica* group, or as fasciolid eggs.

3. *F. buski* is found primarily in the Far East, including Southeast Asia and, especially, Thailand. In infection with *F. buski*, local inflammation occurs when the worms attach to the mucosal wall. Diarrhea and abdominal pain may occur. Eosinophilia is common. Bowel obstruction may result from heavy infections.

4. The pig is the primary reservoir for the giant intestinal fluke. The unembryonated egg is passed in the feces of the pig, dog, rabbit, or human. The miracidium develops within the egg in water in approximately 1 month. The first intermediate host is the snail, which is penetrated by the miracidium. After generation of sporocysts and rediae, cercariae are produced and escape from the snail host. They proceed to encyst, forming metacercariae on freshwater vegetation, including water chestnuts and bamboo.

Humans acquire the infection by the ingestion of encysted metacercariae attached to infected vegetation or after peeling water chestnuts with the teeth. Metacercariae excyst in the small intestine and attach to the jejunal or duodenal wall, where adults develop. Eggs are passed in the stool following cross-fertilization in the intestine.

5. Prevention of infection requires the proper disposal of human fecal waste. The snail population should be markedly reduced to eliminate the first intermediate host, thus interfering with the life cycle.

To prevent many intestinal parasitic infections, the practice of eating raw vegetation should be discouraged or eliminated. Freshwater plants should be boiled for several seconds before being eaten or peeled with the teeth. Use of human fecal waste (night soil) as fertilizer should be discontinued, although in many areas of rural Asia this is not likely to happen.

6. Praziquantel is the drug of choice to treat infections with *F. buski*. Side effects are mild and transient. Niclosamide may be considered as an alternative agent.

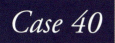

Case 40

The patient was a 66-year-old Hispanic male Vietnam War veteran who had suffered from multiple myeloma for several years and had undergone bone marrow transplantation. He initially appeared to be recovering well following the surgery, but several weeks later he presented to the emergency room with symptoms of diarrhea, cough, dyspnea, and abdominal pain. The patient's pulmonary complaint was diagnosed as chronic obstructive lung disease, and he was treated with high-dose intravenous steroids and inhaled bronchodilators.

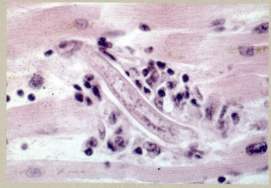

Figure 40.1

One month later, the patient was readmitted with fever and wheezing. At this time he was considered to have exacerbation of his lung disease, as well as congestive heart failure. Blood cultures grew *Enterococcus faecalis* and *Escherichia coli*. Although treated aggressively with antibiotics, the patient's condition deteriorated, and he died 30 days after being readmitted.

A complete autopsy was performed, and microscopic analysis showed nematode larvae in his internal organs, including the heart (Fig. 40.1), small intestine (Fig. 40.2), lungs, and liver. A characteristic larva is shown in Fig. 40.3.

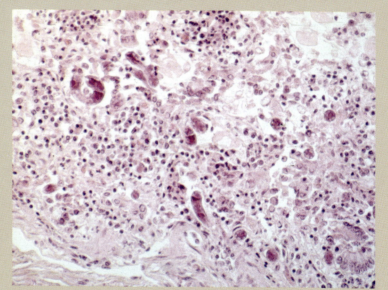

Figure 40.2

QUESTIONS

1. Which intestinal nematodes might have caused this patient's pulmonary symptoms while migrating through the lungs? Which nematode is most probably responsible for the patient's condition?

2. How is the diagnosis of this infection usually made? Which other nematode larvae may be confused with this parasite? How might this happen?

3. Describe the life cycle of this parasite.

4. Which role might the glucocorticoid therapy have played in the severity of this patient's illness?

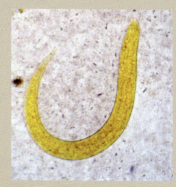

Figure 40.3

5. How might this patient's infection be related to his bone marrow transplant? Discuss the importance of the history of a potential candidate for organ transplantation.

6. In addition to pulmonary symptoms, which other laboratory findings may provide diagnostic aids in determining the etiology of this infection?

7. How is this infection treated?

ANSWERS

1. Nematodes which migrate through the lungs as part of their life cycles include *Ascaris lumbricoides, Strongyloides stercoralis,* and the hookworms *Necator americanus* and *Ancylostoma duodenale. S. stercoralis* is most probably the parasite causing this patient's infection (strongyloidiasis).

2. The diagnosis of strongyloidiasis is usually made by detection of the larvae in stool specimens submitted for ova and parasite examination. Eggs of this parasite are rarely seen. Hookworm larvae are morphologically similar to those of *S. stercoralis.* If a stool specimen is left at room temperature, hookworm eggs may hatch, releasing larvae. It is important to carefully search for hookworm eggs if nematode larvae are suspected of being those of hookworms.

Specialized concentration procedures, such as the use of the Baermann funnel, and cultures (Harada-Mori or petri dish) may prove to be more effective than traditional fecal examinations.

Another method which provides greater sensitivity than direct microscopic examination is the agar culture method. In this procedure, stool is placed on an agar plate and the plate is sealed and held for 2 days at room temperature. As the larvae crawl across the agar, they carry fecal bacteria with them. This results in visible tracks along their paths. The plates are examined under the microscope for larvae. The presence of *S. stercoralis* larvae may be confirmed by washing the plate with 10% formalin and examining a wet preparation of the sediment from the formalin washings.

By using the Entero-Test procedure, duodenal contents may be obtained and examined for the presence of larvae. In disseminated infections, larvae are occasionally identified in sputum specimens.

3. The filariform larvae of *S. stercoralis* are usually found in fecally contaminated soil. These infective larvae penetrate the skin. They then pass into the circulation and migrate to the right heart, lungs, trachea, and pharynx. The larvae are swallowed and mature to adult worms in the intestine in approximately 2 weeks. The female adult worms produce eggs, which usually hatch, releasing rhabditiform larvae in the intestine. These noninfective larvae are usually passed in the feces. In the soil, they develop into infective filariform larvae, ready to penetrate the skin of a new host. In the indirect cycle, the rhabditiform larvae develop into free-living adult males and females, which may live and produce eggs in the soil.

The rhabditiform larvae may develop into the infective filariform larvae in the intestine and may lead to autoinfection. Larvae may infect the host by penetrating the intestinal wall and migrating to the lungs or by passing out of the intestine in the stool and penetrating the perianal skin. Autoinfection often results in disseminated infection and the hyperinfection syndrome.

4. The immunosuppressive effects of intravenous steroids such as glucocorticoids may have resulted in reactivation of a latent infection with this parasite. Dissemination of infection, resulting in the hyperinfection syndrome, with large numbers of larvae being produced, is known to occur in immunocompromised patients. This may have been responsible for the worsening of this patient's symptoms, leading to his deteriorating condition and death.

5. Transplant recipients usually receive high doses of immunosuppressive therapy. This allows the worm burden to greatly increase, sometimes leading to disseminated infection with *S. stercoralis*. It is imperative to rule out the presence of *S. stercoralis* in patients who are to receive organ transplants or immunosuppressive therapy, especially those suffering from diarrhea and abdominal pain and patients from Latin America, in order to prevent serious sequelae. Potential candidates for organ transplantation must be carefully screened for evidence of infection with this parasite before immunosuppressive therapy begins.

6. Eosinophilia often occurs in parasitic infections. Polymicrobial bacteremia with enteric microorganisms (*Enterococcus faecalis* and *Escherichia coli*) is often associated with strongyloidiasis. Fecal microorganisms are often seeded into the blood, when the larvae migrate from the intestine into the bloodstream. Meningitis caused by enteric bacteria may also occur.

7. Ivermectin and thiabendazole are recommended for the treatment of strongyloidiasis.

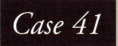

Case 41

A 4-year-old boy was taken to his family practitioner suffering from mild gastrointestinal symptoms, including slight abdominal pain and diarrhea. He had also complained of anal itching. A stool specimen from the patient was submitted for routine culture. The boy's mother was advised to collect three stool specimens on alternate days, to place the stools in vials containing 10% formalin and polyvinyl alcohol fixative, and to submit these specimens to a local hospital laboratory for examination for ova and parasites.

Bacterial cultures were negative for enteric pathogens. Microscopic examination of the concentrated fecal sediments revealed membrane-enclosed packets of helminth eggs (Fig. 41.1). Each packet contained 5 to 30 eggs. Within several eggs, a six-hooked oncosphere was seen. Gravid barrel-shaped proglottids were also observed.

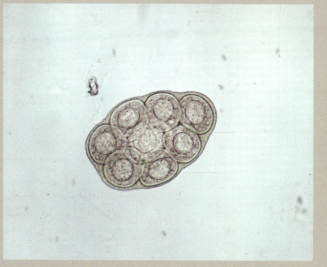

Figure 41.1

QUESTIONS

1. Which cestode do you think is causing this child's symptoms?

2. How would you diagnose this infection?

3. How does the name of this helminth relate to its definitive host? Why is this helminth more common in children than in adults?

4. Describe the life cycle of this helminth.

5. How is this parasite transmitted?

6. Describe the appearance of the proglottids of this helminth.

7. How is this infection treated?

ANSWERS

1. This child is infected with the dog tapeworm, *Dipylidium caninum*.

2. The presence of characteristic gravid proglottids and egg packets (following rupture of proglottids) in human feces is diagnostic for infection with *D. caninum*.

3. *D. caninum* is the most common and widespread adult tapeworm found worldwide in dogs and cats, which act as the definitive hosts. The infection is more common in children, probably because they are more closely associated with dogs and cats and their fleas.

4. Gravid proglottids and egg packets containing multiple oncospheres are passed in the feces of the dog or cat. The proglottids are actively motile and may migrate from the anus of the animal. Eggs are released from the proglottids during a series of contractions. The larval stage of the dog or cat flea acts as the intermediate host by ingesting the eggs and continuing the life cycle. Cysticercoids persist through maturation of the larva to the adult flea. The life cycle is completed when humans accidentally ingest fleas infected with cysticercoid larvae. The larvae develop into adult worms in the small intestine.

5. Infection is initiated after ingestion of *D. caninum* cysticercoid larvae. This is usually a result of accidental hand-to-mouth delivery of adult fleas from infected cats or dogs. Humans (especially children) are infected after accidentally ingesting the fleas.

6. A gravid proglottid is longer than wide and contains two sets of male and female reproductive organs. Proglottids contain compartmentalized packets of 5 to 30 eggs. Proglottids have been described as appearing like cucumber or white watermelon seeds when wet and like rice grains when dry. Oncospheres are sometimes visible in the eggs.

7. A single dose of praziquantel is an effective treatment of infections with *D. caninum* in both children and adults.

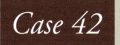

Case 42

A 72-year-old woman from Asia, visiting relatives in the United States, presented to the emergency room suffering from pulmonary symptoms including shortness of breath, cough, and wheezing. She reported having produced a moderate amount of blood-tinged sputum. Several sputum specimens were collected and submitted for bacteriological studies, including routine culture and tuberculosis smear and culture. When the acid-fast smears were reported negative for *Mycobacterium tuberculosis*, a request was submitted for examination of the sputum specimens for ova and parasites. A CBC was also ordered.

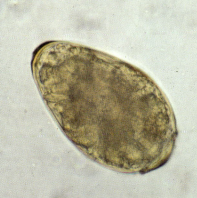

The blood count revealed moderate eosinophilia, with 16% eosinophils. The sputum cultures were negative for routine bacterial pathogens. Examination of the sputum specimen for parasites revealed operculated helminth eggs, characterized by opercular shoulders. A characteristic egg is shown in Fig. 42.1.

Figure 42.1

QUESTIONS

1. Which helminth is causing this patient's symptoms?

2. Which other intestinal helminths may be diagnosed by examination of sputum specimens? Explain.

3. How is the diagnosis of this infection usually made?

4. Which helminth may be confused with this parasite? Why?

5. Describe the life cycle of this helminth.

6. In addition to ingestion of infected food, how else is this infection acquired?

7. How is this infection treated?

ANSWERS

1. The lung fluke, *Paragonimus westermani*, is causing this patient's pulmonary symptoms. Many other species of *Paragonimus* infect humans in many parts of the world. *P. mexicanus* is an important human pathogen in Central and South America. The presence of larvae in the lungs often leads to coughing and hemoptysis, particularly following paroxysms of coughing.

2. In addition to the lung fluke, nematodes which migrate through the lungs as part of their life cycles include *Ascaris lumbricoides*, *Strongyloides stercoralis*, and the hookworms *Necator americanus* and *Ancylostoma duodenale*. During their migration through the lungs, these larvae also may cause pulmonary symptoms and may be recovered from sputum specimens. Eggs are not frequently recovered in sputum unless the patient is symptomatic.

3. Paragonimiasis should be suspected in patients with typical pulmonary symptoms who reside in areas of endemic infection and have a history of eating raw crabs or crayfish. The diagnosis of infection with *P. westermani* may be made by examination of wet preparations of both sputum and fecal specimens. The zinc sulfate flotation method is unsatisfactory for diagnosis, since the operculated eggs do not float. The sedimentation concentration method is preferred. The thick-shelled, unembryonated, ovoid, brownish yellow eggs of this parasite are readily seen microscopically, using the low-power (10×) objective. Multiple specimens may be required to make the diagnosis if the worm burden is low.

4. The operculated ova of *Diphyllobothrium latum*, the broad or fish tapeworm, resemble those of *P. westermani* in size and appearance. However, the ova of tapeworm eggs lack the opercular shoulders present on the eggs of *P. westermani*. The eggshell of the lung fluke also has a thickened abopercular end.

5. Unembryonated eggs are passed in human feces or sputum. Larvae develop in water for about 2 weeks. A miradicium is released and infects a snail, which acts as the first intermediate host. Cercariae develop in the snail. After being released, cercariae infect crayfish or crabs (second intermediate hosts) by passing through the gill chamber. The second intermediate host may also become infected by ingesting the snail. The cercariae encyst in the tissues of the crab or crayfish as metacercariae.

   Humans are accidental hosts and become infected after eating raw or insufficiently cooked crabs or crayfish, which bear encysted metacercariae. Metacercariae excyst in the duodenum. They then migrate through the intestinal wall into the abdominal cavity and through the diaphragm into the pleural cavity and lungs. In the bronchioles, larvae develop into adults, which become encapsulated in the lungs. Eggs are released into the bronchi and may be found in sputum. Eggs may be coughed up and swallowed and may therefore also be found in feces.

6. An individual may become infected by handling or crushing infected crabs or crayfish in preparation for cooking. Metacercariae may then contaminate the fingers, cutting boards, or cooking utensils and be accidentally ingested.

7. Although few patients require therapy, praziquantel is the drug of choice to treat infections with *P. westermani*. Side effects are mild and transient. An alternative agent is bithionol.

Case 43

A 4-year-old boy living in the southeastern United States presented to his family physician suffering from diarrhea, abdominal pain, and nausea. Blood was drawn for analysis and revealed a hemoglobin level of 12 g/dl. A culture for bacterial pathogens was ordered, and three stool specimens were submitted for ova and parasite examinations.

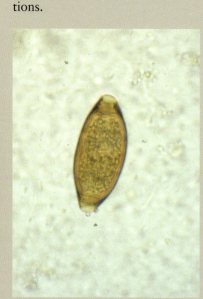

Figure 43.1

The bacterial culture was negative for enteric pathogens. Microscopic analysis of concentrated sediments of the stool specimens revealed numerous bile-stained, barrel-shaped nematode eggs. The eggs were characterized by having clear, prominent polar plugs. A characteristic egg is shown in Fig. 43.1.

QUESTIONS

1. Which helminth ova would fit the description of those seen in the patient's stool specimen?

2. Describe the appearance of the adult worm, which explains the common name of this nematode.

3. Describe the life cycle of this parasite.

4. How is the diagnosis of this infection made? How does the patient's blood test results relate to his infection?

5. How is infection with this parasite prevented?

6. How is this infection treated?

ANSWERS

1. The bile-stained, barrel-shaped ova with prominent polar plugs at each end, shown in Fig. 43.1, most closely resemble those of the nematode *Trichuris trichiura*.

2. The nematode is referred to as the whipworm because the adult worm resembles a whip. This nematode has a long, slender, threadlike anterior portion and a thicker posterior portion with the appearance of a whip handle. The adult male worm is smaller than the female and has a coiled tail.

3. *T. trichiura* has a direct life cycle. Human infection with *T. trichiura* is acquired by the ingestion of soil containing embryonated eggs. Eggs are passed in the feces. After approximately 2 weeks in moist soil, the eggs become mature, and at this time they are infective. Embryonated eggs contain first-stage larvae and are ingested from contaminated soil by humans. The shell is digested in the small intestine. The worms develop in the duodenum and cecum. They attach by insinuating their slender anterior ends into the intestinal mucosal epithelium. In about 3 months, the adult worm begins to lay eggs.

4. Whipworm infections are usually easily diagnosed by the detection of characteristic eggs (as seen in Fig. 43.1) in a permanent stain or, more commonly, in a wet preparation or concentrated stool sediment. Eggs should be counted, since light infections may not require treatment.

   Adult worms are rarely found in the stool, since they are attached to the intestinal wall. Serious *T. trichiura* infection in children may result in blood loss, leading to anemia, a symptom found in this patient.

5. Prevention of infection requires adherence to good personal hygiene practices and avoidance of contaminated food or water, as well as the avoidance of using human feces as fertilizer.

6. Mebendazole and albendazole are effective drugs to treat whipworm infection. Although it may not be necessary to treat well-nourished children, undernourished children might show cognitive improvement with treatment.

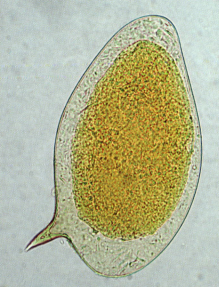

Case 44

A young African woman was visiting American relatives and developed fever, malaise, a rash, diarrhea, and abdominal pain. Her relatives brought her to the family doctor for examination. She was noted to have liver tenderness. Blood was drawn for CBC and liver enzyme analysis. A stool specimen was submitted for bacterial culture, and three stool specimens were sent for ova and parasite examination.

The patient was noted to be mildly anemic and had slightly elevated liver enzyme levels. The culture was negative for bacterial pathogens. Two of the three stool specimens revealed a small number of helminth eggs; the third specimen was negative for parasites. Each oval, light-yellow–brown egg measured approximately 170 by 70 μm and was characterized by having a prominent lateral spine projecting from one side. A typical egg is shown in Fig. 44.1.

Figure 44.1

QUESTIONS

1. Which helminth is causing this patient's infection?

2. How is this infection diagnosed? How is hatching used to determine egg viability?

3. Describe the appearance of the ova of this parasite. How do these ova compare with those of other members of this genus?

4. Describe the life cycle of this helminth.

5. What is Katayama fever?

6. How does this helminth differ from other human trematodes?

7. Do bird helminths in this genus cause human disease?

8. How is this infection treated?

ANSWERS

1. The helminth causing this patient's infection is the blood fluke, *Schistosoma mansoni*.

2. The diagnosis of infection with *S. mansoni* is made by the detection of characteristic eggs in stool specimens. Eggs can be detected only after the worms mature, which may take 4 to 7 weeks after infection. Eggs can easily be distinguished from those of *S. japonicum*, which are also found in fecal specimens. Viable miracidia are sometimes observed in the fecal preparation of a fresh nonpreserved specimen. Multiple stool specimens may need to be examined if the patient has a low worm burden. Travel history may be helpful in the diagnosis of schistosomiasis.

Hatching tests may be used in the diagnosis of chronic schistosomiasis to determine egg viability when the worm burden is light. The test is designed to mimic conditions in nature, with spring water and sunlight. For a description of the test, see case 34.

3. The eggs of *S. mansoni* are oval and are a light yellow-brown color. Each egg is up to 180 μm in length and up to 73 μm in width, with a well-developed lateral spine. The eggs of *S. haematobium* have a similar shape but are smaller and have a prominent terminal spine. The smallest eggs, which measure up to 100 μm in length and up to 65 μm in width, are those of *S. japonicum*; each egg is round and has an often unrecognizable small, lateral spine.

4. Free-swimming cercariae penetrate human skin. After entering the host, the parasite is called a schistosomulum. The schistosome cercariae lose their bifurcated tails following skin penetration. These forms enter the circulation, mature in the portal blood, enter the blood vessels, and are carried to the lungs, intestinal tract, and liver. The worms mature to the adult form in the sinusoids of the liver. The adults then migrate to the venules of the inferior mesenteric veins, where eggs are laid and extruded into the lumen of the intestine. These eggs are immature when first laid and develop a miracidium in 8 to 10 days.

The eggs leave the body in feces. The miracidium is mature when it is released from the egg in water. It finds and penetrates a suitable snail host. Cercariae are produced and released from the snail into the water.

5. Katayama fever is the name given to acute schistosomiasis. It is named for the area of Japan where it was first recognized. This type of infection occurs when the primary infection is heavy and egg production begins. The symptoms include an abrupt onset of chills, fever, hepatosplenomegaly, dysentery, and eosinophilia and tend to be quite severe. This illness occurs a few weeks following initial infection, and mortality is high.

6. Schistosomes, or blood flukes, differ from other human trematodes in that they have two sexes, which differ in appearance. Female worms are long, slender, and cylindrical, while male worms are shorter and somewhat flattened. The blood flukes reside in blood vessels.

The eggs of schistosomes lack the operculum seen in the eggs of other trematodes. The eggs rupture on exposure to water. Most trematode infections are acquired by ingestion of encysted metacercariae. No metacercarial stage exists in the life cycles of schistosomes. Cercariae, which have forked tails, are found in water and directly penetrate human skin.

7. Nonhuman schistosomes, such as bird schistosomes, are unable to complete their life cycles in humans and die without maturing. Following skin penetration, the cercariae migrate in human skin and die in the subcutaneous tissues, eliciting immediate hypersensitivity reactions in the human host. This condition is known by several names, including swimmer's itch, clam digger's itch, schistosome dermatitis, and cercarial dermatitis. Symptoms vary due to host susceptibility and previous exposure. Humans become infected while swimming in contaminated water. Any body of water harboring infected snails may result in cercarial dermatitis.

8. Praziquantel is the drug of choice to treat infections with *S. mansoni,* although the drug is ineffective against immature stages of schistosomes. A single oral dose is usually adequate for treatment and has mild and transient side effects. Oxamniquine is also effective against American and West African strains of *S. mansoni;* North and East African strains are less sensitive to this agent, and a higher dose over a 2- to 3-day period is required.

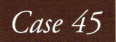

Case 45

A 9-year-old boy was taken to his pediatrician with a headache and gastrointestinal symptoms, including abdominal pain and persistent diarrhea. He had experienced a 3-lb weight loss over several weeks and had little appetite. A stool sample was sent immediately to the laboratory for bacterial analysis and examination for ova and parasites.

The specimen showed no evidence of bacterial pathogens, but oval, thin-shelled helminth eggs were seen microscopically in the fresh specimen (Fig. 45.1). Oncospheres having numerous polar filaments were observed in the eggs. A proglottid containing eggs is shown in Fig. 45.2.

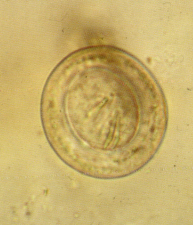

Figure 45.1

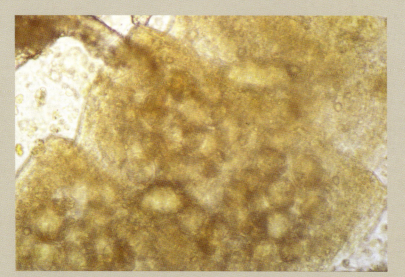

Figure 45.2

QUESTIONS

1. Which helminth is causing this patient's symptoms?

2. Why is this helminth unusual among members of its class?

3. How is this helminth transmitted?

4. How is the diagnosis of this infection made?

5. Describe the life cycle of this helminth.

6. How is this infection treated?

ANSWERS

1. The patient is infected with *Hymenolepis nana*. This helminth is a cestode and is the smallest tapeworm known to infect humans. It is known as the dwarf tapeworm.

2. This tapeworm is unusual among cestodes because no intermediate host is required to complete the life cycle. Frequently found in mice and other rodents, which act as reservoirs of infection, *H. nana* is the most common tapeworm found in the United States.

3. Infection with *H. nana* usually begins with ingestion of infective eggs. Eggs hatch in the small intestine. A six-hooked oncosphere develops into a cysticercoid larva. The larva matures into the adult worm (see life cycle). No intermediate host is required to complete the life cycle, but larvae may develop in intermediate hosts such as beetles (especially grain beetles) or fleas. Although ingestion of beetles found in grain or cereals may transport the larvae into the human host, this mechanism of infection is uncommon.

4. Diagnosis of infection with *H. nana* is usually made by the recovery of characteristic round to oval thin-shelled eggs in human feces. Fresh specimens are preferred. If preserved specimens are received, formalin-based fixatives are recommended over polyvinyl alcohol. Each egg contains two polar thickenings or knobs, from which four to eight polar filaments arise. The eggs of *H. diminuta* resemble those of *H. nana* without the polar filaments but are larger.

   Adult worms and proglottids are rarely seen in the stool. When seen in stained specimens, *H. nana* proglottids resemble those of *H. diminuta*. The saclike gravid uterus is usually full of eggs and fills most of the uterine cavity. Eggs are discharged continually until the proglottid detaches and is excreted or undergoes decomposition.

5. After ingestion, the eggs hatch in the stomach or small intestine. The released oncospheres (larvae) penetrate the small intestinal wall and develop into the cysticercoid stage in tissue. The cysticercoid larvae migrate back into the small intestine and mature. The scolex attaches to the mucosa, where the adult tapeworm resides and reproduces. Eggs are released when the gravid proglottids disintegrate. Eggs, which are infective when passed, leave the body in feces. They may be ingested by humans or by other animal hosts, which become infected when the cysticercoid larvae develop. Eggs sometimes hatch in the intestine. The resulting cysticercoid larvae may develop to adulthood and often result in autoinfection.

6. Praziquantel and niclosamide are effective in treating infections with *H. nana*.

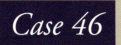

A 68-year-old man from a sheep-rearing area of the People's Republic of China had moved to the United States to live with his son. He visited his son's physician for a routine physical examination. His physician noted an enlarged liver, with a palpable mass in the right upper quadrant of the abdomen.

Radiology studies were ordered, and a round space-occupying lesion was demonstrated in the liver. Microscopic examination of a biopsy specimen confirmed the diagnosis of a parasitic infection (Fig. 46.1). During a surgical procedure to remove the hepatic cyst, aspiration of the cyst contents was performed and the contents were also examined microscopically.

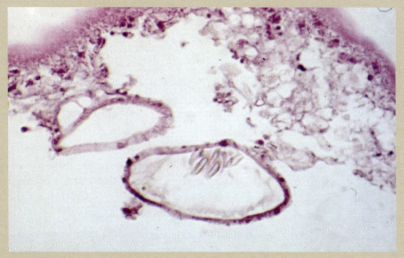

Figure 46.1

QUESTIONS

1. Based on the patient's symptoms, which parasitic infection do you think he has?

2. What aspect of the patient's history is a clue to his infection?

3. Describe the nature of the patient's hepatic cyst.

4. What danger to the patient exists during surgical removal and aspiration of the cyst?

5. Describe the life cycle of this helminth.

6. How would you treat this patient?

ANSWERS

1. Based on the patient's symptoms of an enlarged liver, an abdominal mass in the right quadrant of the abdomen, and the biopsy specimen shown in Fig. 46.1, he probably has liver hydatid cyst disease caused by *Echinococcus granulosus*. Although not routinely performed, the aspiration of cyst fluid is sometimes used in the diagnosis of this infection. Microscopic examination of the aspirated cyst fluid probably detected the presence of hydatid sand, a granular material consisting of free scolices, free cysts, and amorphous germinal material.

2. The patient was from a sheep-rearing area of China, where hydatid cyst disease is endemic. This infection is a major health problem in this part of the world.

3. A hydatid cyst, which may become very large, has a thick, laminated outer layer and an inner layer of germinal epithelial tissue from which the daughter cysts and brood capsules (smaller cysts containing several developing inverted scolices) bud into the cavity of the cyst. Daughter cysts are tiny replicas of the hydatid cyst itself, with the laminated outer layer. The cyst also contains hydatid sand (described above). Some cysts are sterile and contain no sand. There is also a great deal of fluid inside the cyst.

4. During the surgical removal and aspiration of a hydatid cyst, fluid or tissue may leak out into the peritoneal cavity. Hydatid sand or bits of tissue may produce new cysts and cause disseminated infection. Anaphylactic shock may also occur.

5. A dog or other definitive canine host becomes infected with *E. granulosus* by eating raw viscera containing parasite cysts from slaughtered infected livestock (intermediate hosts) such as sheep. Scolices from hydatid cysts attach to the mucosa of the small intestine. Adult worms develop. Eggs and proglottids are passed in the dog's feces and are ingested by humans or herbivores such as sheep. The eggs hatch, penetrate the intestinal wall, enter the circulation, and are carried to tissues, forming hydatid cysts in organs, especially the liver and lungs.

6. Surgery is considered the treatment of choice in treating hydatid cyst disease if the patient has a unilocular cyst in an operable body region. Hydatid liver cysts have been treated with a cutting aspiration device. This is apparently a safe and effective procedure. As alternative treatments, mebendazole and albendazole have been used.

REFERENCES

Garcia, L. S. 2001. *Diagnostic Medical Parasitology,* 4th ed., p. 265–295. ASM Press, Washington, D.C.

Heelan, J. S., and F. W. Ingersoll. 2002. *Essentials of Human Parasitology,* p. 138–149. Thomson Delmar Learning, Albany, N.Y.

Markell, E. K., D. T. John, and W. A. Krotoski. 1999. *Markell and Voge's Medical Parasitology,* 8th ed., p. 269–303. The W. B. Saunders Co., Philadelphia, Pa.

Zeibig, E. A. 1997. *Clinical Parasitology,* p. 128–163. The W. B. Saunders Co., Philadelphia, Pa.

This section includes cases of infection with slender, threadlike nematodes known as filarial worms or filariae, as well as other tissue nematodes or roundworms. These helminths are transmitted by the bite of arthropod vectors. Vectors include biting insects such as flies and mosquitoes. Specific filarial infections occur in geographical areas inhabited by specific vectors. The filarial nematodes live in the lymphatic systems or the subcutaneous or deep connective tissue of the host. They produce larvae known as microfilariae, which circulate in the blood and lymphatic system. These larvae, in adapting to the feeding habits of their vectors, exhibit periodicity, appearing in the blood only at certain times of the day.

Filariae that cause lymphatic filariasis, often called elephantiasis, include *Brugia malayi* (brugian filariasis) and *Wuchereria bancrofti* (Bancroftian filariasis). The filariae causing lymphatic filariasis are diagnosed by the preparation and examination of lymphatic fluid smears or thin and thick peripheral blood films for microfilariae. Concentration techniques, using centrifugation or filtration methods, may be useful in making a diagnosis in light infections. Microfilariae, although not demonstrable in all patients, are characteristic for each of the filariae and may be used in the identification of the worm. Characteristics of the microfilariae useful in the identification of these parasites include the presence or absence of a membrane or sheath, the shape and size of the larva, and the arrangement of body nuclei in the tail. Hematology studies may be useful to detect eosinophilia, often associated with filarial infections.

Although surgical procedures are sometimes recommended, a number of antimicrobial agents are available to treat infections with lymphatic filarial nematodes.

Loa loa is a filarial worm that causes loiasis. Adult worms inhabit the subcutaneous or deep tissues and may be seen crossing the conjunctiva of the eye. Characteristic microfilariae may be seen in thick and thin peripheral blood smears, but often not for years after infection. Therefore, knowledge of the patient's travel history or residential area provides useful information and is particularly important in making the diagnosis of loiasis. Although surgical intervention may be indicated, drugs are available to treat this infection.

Onchocerca volvulus is a filarial nematode that causes onchocerciasis (river blindness). This infection is of economic concern, as well as a major public health problem. Adult worms become encapsulated within fibrous nodules, and ocular lesions may lead to blindness. This infection may be diagnosed by the microscopic examination of a skin biopsy specimen or "skin snip," which may be placed in saline and teased to reveal microfilariae or cultured and examined after a while.

Worms may be surgically removed, although drugs are available to treat onchocerciasis.

Trichinella spiralis, or the trichina worm, causes trichinosis, now rare in the United States. This parasite is commonly found in wild and domestic mammals; transmission of infection usually occurs by the ingestion of raw or poorly cooked infected meat. The larvae usually encyst in striated muscle tissue of the reservoir host. Humans are accidental hosts, in whom larvae encyst in striated skeletal muscle tissue. Trichinosis is usually diagnosed by the demonstration of larvae in a muscle biopsy specimen. Drugs are available to treat patients with trichinosis.

The guinea worm, *Dracunculus medinensis,* causes dracunculiasis and is a public health problem in some parts of the world, such as Africa. Vectors for this worm are tiny crustaceans known as copepods. Human infection occurs following ingestion of drinking water contaminated with infected copepods. Dracunculiasis is usually diagnosed clinically or by the recognition of the characteristic worm-containing lesion associated with this infection. The worm may be manually removed, or drugs may be used to treat this infection.

Baylisascaris procyonis, the raccoon ascarid, causes a recently recognized helminthic zoonotic infection known as baylisascariasis. Infections, which may be fatal, occur after the accidental ingestion of the eggs of this worm. Larva migrans may occur in different parts of the body, including the central nervous system. Infections, although rare, are most common in young children. No effective cure is known for this infection.

Nematodes in the family Anisakidae may cause human infection following the ingestion of insufficiently cooked saltwater fish or squid. A history of eating fish is helpful in making the diagnosis of anisakiasis. The worm is sometimes seen during gastroscopic examination. Treatment is not usually necessary for this infection, unless worms embed in the stomach wall.

Toxocara canis is a nematode found in dogs, especially puppies. The infection is transmitted, often to young children, following the accidental ingestion of infective eggs of the worm. The infection manifests itself as visceral larva migrans; larvae do not develop into adults but migrate in different parts of the body. Although drugs are available to treat this infection, the disease may be self-limited.

Case 47

An 18-year-old male refugee from West Africa was seen by a family practitioner in the United States for fever and facial pain. On physical examination, peripheral edema was noted.

Blood was drawn for laboratory studies. Eosinophilia (30%) was present. Examination of a Giemsa-stained peripheral blood smear revealed the presence of a moderate number of sheathed microfilariae averaging 250 μm in length. Some of the sheaths stained poorly, appearing as "halos" around the organisms. Microfilariae were concentrated at the edges of the blood smear. Nuclei in the microfilariae extended in a continuous row to the tips of tails. A sheathed microfilaria is shown in Fig. 47.1.

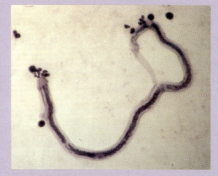

Figure 47.1

QUESTIONS

1. Which nematode is causing this patient's symptoms?

2. Calabar swellings are often noted in these patients. What are they?

3. What are microfilariae?

4. Describe the life cycle of this parasite.

5. How does the morphological appearance of the microfilariae allow identification of the nematode causing the infection?

6. How is this infection diagnosed? Why did the microfilariae in this patient's blood stain poorly? Does the appearance of a "halo" always indicate a sheath?

7. Discuss the treatment of this infection.

ANSWERS

1. The patient has loiasis, caused by the African eye worm, *Loa loa*. This helminth is one of a group of long, threadlike nematodes called filariae which parasitize humans. The adult worm is known to migrate through subcutaneous tissue and across the eye.

2. Calabar (fugitive) swellings, named for the Nigerian town where they were initially reported, are localized patches of subcutaneous edema which may appear anywhere on the body but most frequently occur on the extremities. They result from an inflammatory reaction caused by the presence of either the worms or the metabolic by-products of the worms. They develop rapidly over a few hours and usually last for a few days before subsiding gradually. They may, however, last for several weeks. Itchiness and pain usually preceed the development of these swellings. The adult worm is not necessarily present near the Calabar swelling when it develops.

3. Female filariae produce microfilariae, which are highly motile, thread-like pre-larvae that circulate in the bloodstream. They may or may not possess a sheath, depending on whether they retain (sheathed form) or rupture (unsheathed form) the egg membrane. The shape and size of the microfilariae allow them to exist within the vascular system or migrate through tissues. Microfilariae may live for a long period in the vertebrate host.

4. Female *L. loa* worms produce sheathed microfilariae, which circulate in the bloodstream. Microfilariae are ingested by the mango fly or the deer fly during a blood meal and develop into infective larvae. Larvae migrate to the mouth parts of the fly. The infective larvae are deposited on a person's skin and actively migrate into the wound when the fly bites. The larvae develop to maturity in subcutaneous tissue. Male and female adult worms migrate in subcutaneous tissue, in deep connective tissue, in the skin, and beneath the conjunctiva. Adult male worms are 20 to 35 mm long; the females are slightly longer, ranging in size from 50 to 70 mm. Calabar swellings are due to angioedema.

   Adult worms migrating through the subcutaneous tissue usually cause no discomfort to the patient and are generally noticeable only when migrating through the conjunctiva or across the bridge of the nose.

5. Microfilariae produced by different filariae may be identified by the presence or absence of a sheath and may also be distinguished by their size and the arrangement of nuclei in the tail.

6. The diagnosis of loiasis may be made by microscopic examination of Giemsa or hematoxylin stains (such as Delafield's hematoxylin) of thick and thin smears of peripheral blood. The microfilariae may stain poorly and not be identified correctly in routine blood films, since Giemsa stain does not stain the microfilarial sheath adequately; hematoxylin stains do provide adequate staining. The appearance of "halos" around the microfilariae does not always indicate the presence of a sheath. This effect might be due to shrinkage.

The Knott concentration technique and filtration of blood through a Nuclepore filter are also useful techniques to make this diagnosis. In the Knott technique, up to 1 ml of blood per 10 ml of 2% formalin is concentrated. The sediment may be examined as a wet preparation or stained for microfilariae. In the Nuclepore method, polycarbonate filters are used to trap microfilariae after red blood cells are lysed. The filter may be examined directly on a microscope slide.

A history of Calabar swellings and the presence of eosinophilia aid in the diagnosis. Sheathed microfilariae of *L. loa* are 250 to 300 μm long, with rounded anterior ends and a continuous row of nuclei extending to the tip of the tail. They have a diurnal periodicity, with a peak worm burden at midday. Blood samples for the diagnosis of loiasis should therefore be collected during the daytime hours. However, since the microfilariae often do not appear in the patient's blood until years after the adult worms or the host reaction to infection is noted, the diagnosis is frequently made by reviewing the medical history or the patient's history of travel to or residence in an area of endemic infection. The worms are occasionally detected while migrating across the bridge of the nose or across the conjunctiva.

7. The usual treatment for loiasis is diethylcarbamazine, but side reactions may occur if the worm burden is high. Neurological complications are the most serious sequelae resulting from treatment. Ivermectin and albendazole have also been effective in reducing microfilaremia. Although not routinely performed, surgical removal of the adult worms is relatively simple and may be performed during the worm's migration across the conjunctiva or the bridge of the nose.

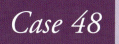

Case 48

A 26-year-old Nigerian man who was attending graduate school in the United States had spent the afternoon swimming with friends. He later presented to the college infirmary with symptoms of nausea, vomiting, urticaria, and severe itching. He also complained of a painful blister-like ulcer on his foot. The ulcer had a reddish color and was approximately 6 cm in diameter. The examining physician noted what appeared to be a worm protruding from the ulcer.

QUESTIONS

1. Which worm is causing this patient's infection? What is the name of the infection?

2. How is this infection acquired?

3. Describe the life cycle of this helminth.

4. Which other conditions might be confused with this infection?

5. What is the traditional method of removing this worm? What is the inherent risk in this procedure? Which drugs are available to treat this infection?

6. What kinds of efforts have been made to control the spread of this infection?

ANSWERS

1. The worm protruding from the ulcer and causing the patient's infection is the guinea worm, *Dracunculus medinensis*. The infection is known as dracunculiasis, dracunculosis, or dracontiasis.

2. The infection is acquired by the ingestion of drinking water containing the intermediate hosts, which are copepods in the genus *Cyclops*. Transmission of dracunculiasis requires a body of water where *Cyclops* breeds, direct contact between infected individuals and these bodies of water, and the use of this contaminated water for drinking. Sources of contaminated drinking water vary in different parts of the world and include shallow wells, ponds, and human-made water holes. In India, step wells are a common source of infection. Covered cisterns in Iran and ponds in Ghana serve as reservoirs of infection in those areas.

3. In the human host, larvae are released in the stomach and pass through the wall of the duodenum, through the peritoneal cavity, and into the abdomen and thorax. Worms mature in the deep connective tissue. After mating, gravid females, whose uteri contain numerous rhabditiform larvae, migrate to the subcutaneous tissues. The smaller, inconspicuous males remain in the tissues, become encapsulated, and die.

About 1 year after infection (perhaps earlier), the mature female moves to the skin, where a papule is produced. In a few days, the papule develops into a blister-like ulcer. When the affected body part, often the foot or ankle, is immersed in water, the prolapsed uterus of the worm releases large numbers of first-stage rhabditiform larvae. This process may occur several times. After release of the larvae, the female worm may be extruded from the body or may withdraw to deeper tissues, where it eventually becomes resorbed. The larvae are actively motile and survive for several days in the water.

The rhabditiform larvae are ingested by copepods, where they develop into the infective larvae in about 2 weeks.

4. The lesions found in dracunculiasis may be confused with carbuncles, deep cellulitis, focal myositis, or periostitis.

5. The traditional method for removal of *D. medinensis* is to slowly wind the worm around a stick, a few centimeters a day. Metronidazole is often used to complement or replace the traditional removal of the worm. Other available drugs include niridazole, thiabendazole, and mebendazole.

The inherent risk in this procedure is breaking of the worm during the extraction process. Great skill is necessary for the extraction, since the worm has a very thin body wall and may easily rupture if stretched. An intense inflammatory reaction may occur in these cases. Secondary infection very commonly develops following these events and is a major problem in dracunculiasis.

6. As mentioned above, the transmission of dracunculiasis is dependent on the presence of *Cyclops* copepods in the water, access to this body of water by infected humans, and use of this water source for drinking. Interventions to halt this transmission have evolved on several levels. The World Health Organization has made tremendous efforts to eradicate this infection and to provide a safe water supply to areas where the infection is endemic. These efforts have been very successful and, while not eliminating this infection entirely, have reduced the prevalence of infection in most areas except for India, Pakistan, and a few countries in Africa, especially Sudan and Ghana. Some of the remaining obstacles to complete eradication of the guinea worm include internal strife and civil wars in Africa and apathy of some officials.

Filtration of drinking water using ordinary cloth filters placed over pipes to remove infected *Cyclops* copepods has contributed to reducing the rate of infection in some rural villages. One effective technique based on this method is to attach the filter material to the end of a piece of plastic pipe, much like a straw, and use the pipe to drink directly from the water.

Identifying actively infected patients and preventing them from using town water supplies for bathing purposes has been employed effectively to reduce the spread of dracunculiasis. Vector control using methods to remove or kill *Cyclops* were initially considered to be impractical, since the levels of toxic chemicals needed to effect the killing made the water undrinkable. Even when more recently discovered, safer insecticides are used, this approach is expensive and has met with limited success.

Health education, both in using cloth filters and in preventing contamination of drinking-water sources, has been highly effective in controlling the spread of this disease.

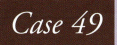

Case 49 A 39-year-old man from Samoa was living and studying in the United States. He presented to the emergency department with fever, lymphadenitis, and lymphangitis. Lymphedema was noted in his extremities and in his scrotum. The patient's symptoms, combined with his geographical area of origin, created a suspicion of a parasitic infection. Blood was sent to the laboratory for a complete blood count and thick and thin smears.

Eosinophilia (30%) was present. Smears were stained by Delafield's hematoxylin method and examined microscopically. A moderate number of sheathed microfilariae averaging 270 μm in length, with bluntly rounded anterior portions, were revealed. A large number of distinct nuclei were seen in the microfilariae; nuclei did not extend to the tips of the tails, which tapered to a point. A sheathed microfilaria is shown in Fig. 49.1.

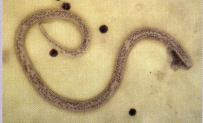

Figure 49.1

QUESTIONS

1. Which nematode is causing this patient's symptoms?

2. How is this nematode distinguished from related helminths?

3. Which insects act as the intermediate hosts for this parasite?

4. Describe the life cycle of this parasite.

5. How is the diagnosis of this infection made? Why was Delafield's hematoxylin stain used?

6. Which drugs may be used to treat this infection?

ANSWERS

1. The patient has filariasis and is infected with *Wuchereria bancrofti,* a filarial nematode that causes lymphatic filariasis. Infection with this nematode is of interest, since it was the first parasitic infection known to be transmitted by an arthropod vector.

2. The microfilariae of *W. bancrofti* are sheathed, with bluntly rounded anterior ends, and measure 245 to 300 μm in length. They have numerous nuclei which do not extend to the tip of the tail; the tail tapers to a point. The sheathed microfilariae of *Brugia malayi,* which also causes lymphatic filariasis, have nuclei, which extend to the tip of the tail; the two terminal nuclei are clearly set apart from the others.

3. The intermediate hosts for *W. bancrofti* are mosquitoes in the genera *Aedes,* *Anopheles,* and *Culex.*

4. Female *W. bancrofti* worms produce sheathed microfilariae which circulate in the bloodstream. Microfilariae are ingested by a mosquito during a blood meal. The microfilariae lose their sheaths (which are digested away in the stomach of the mosquito), penetrate the stomach wall, enter the body cavity of the insect, and migrate to the thoracic muscles. Here they develop into infective larvae and migrate to the proboscis of the mosquito.

The infective larvae leave the proboscis of the mosquito and are deposited on a person's skin. They actively migrate into the wound when the mosquito bites. The larvae enter the peripheral lymphatics and migrate to lymph nodes and lymph vessels. Here they mature to adult male and female worms, which mate. Adult male worms average 40 mm; the females are slightly longer, measuring 80 to 100 mm. Microfilariae are produced after mating and are released from the gravid females.

5. The diagnosis of lymphatic filariasis caused by *W. bancrofti* is made by the microscopic examination of Giemsa- or Delafield's hematoxylin-stained thick and thin blood smears for the morphologically characteristic microfilariae produced by this nematode. Giemsa stain does not stain the microfilarial sheath adequately; hematoxylin does provide adequate staining. Prolonged standing in anticoagulated blood often causes the microfilaria to lose its sheath, leading to difficulties in identification.

The use of the Knott concentration technique or filtration of blood through a Nuclepore filter may aid in the diagnosis of this infection (for details of these techniques, see case 47). In many areas of the world where bancroftian filariasis is endemic, microfilariae exhibit nocturnal periodicity, whereby microfilariae are present in the largest numbers during the night. To detect these infections, blood for thick and thin smears should be drawn between 10 p.m. and 4 a.m. Subperiodic periodicity is characteristic of bancroftian filariasis from Samoa and throughout the Pacific islands. Persons exhibiting this type of illness exhibit microfilaremia at all times, particularly between noon and 8 p.m.

6. The usual treatment of filariasis is diethylcarbamazine or ivermectin. These drugs may be used in combination with albendazole. Diethylcarbamazine, which may be given orally, rapidly kills microfilariae and can kill some adult worms. Treatment is usually spaced over months to years rather than in a more concentrated fashion. Side effects include fever, urticaria, and lymphangitis and are probably due to destruction of the microfilariae and adult worms. Ivermectin may also be taken orally and may be used alone, or in combination with diethylcarbamazine.

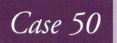

Case 50

A 29-year-old Asian woman, who had moved to the United States a year previously to live with relatives, began to complain of swelling in her right leg below the knee. The patient's relatives took her to a walk-in clinic, where she was examined. The examining physician found enlarged lymph nodes in her right leg. Based on the patient's clinical symptoms and the fact that she had lived in Asia before coming to the United States, he suspected a parasitic infection and ordered thick and thin blood smears.

Blood was collected, and thick and thin smears were prepared. They were stained by the Giemsa method and examined for parasites. Microfilariae were identified in the smears (Fig. 50.1), and a diagnosis of elephantiasis was made. Nuclei were seen extending to the tip of the tails of the sheathed microfilariae, and the two terminal tail nuclei were set apart from the others.

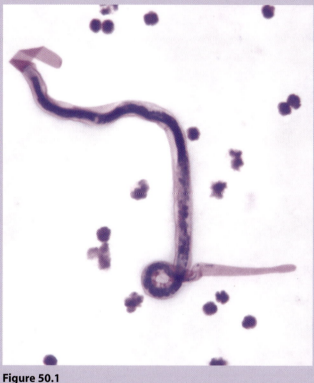

Figure 50.1

QUESTIONS

1. Name the filarial nematode which is causing this patient's infection.

2. How are the microfilariae of this nematode distinguished from those of related helminths?

3. Describe the life cycle of this parasite.

4. How is the diagnosis of this infection made?

5. How is this infection treated?

ANSWERS

1. The diagnosis was based on the appearance of the microfilariae seen in the blood smears. This patient is infected with the filarial nematode *Brugia malayi*.

2. The microfilariae of *B. malayi* are sheathed and measure 175 to 230 μm in length. They have nuclei which extend to the tip of the tail, and the two terminal nuclei are clearly set apart from the others. The nucleus at the tip of the tail is quite small. The microfilariae of *Wuchereria bancrofti* have numerous nuclei which do not extend to the tip of the tail. The tails of both microfilariae taper to a point.

3. Female *B. malayi* worms produce sheathed microfilariae, which circulate in the bloodstream and are ingested by a mosquito during a blood meal. The microfilariae lose their sheaths, penetrate the stomach wall, enter the body cavity of the insect, and migrate to the thoracic muscles. Here they develop into infective larvae and migrate to the proboscis of the mosquito.

   The infective larvae leave the proboscis of the mosquito and are deposited on a person's skin. They actively migrate into the wound when the mosquito bites. The larvae enter the peripheral lymphatics and migrate to lymph nodes and lymph vessels. Here they mature to adult male and female worms, which mate. Microfilariae are produced after mating and are released from the gravid females.

   The life cycles of *B. malayi* and *W. bancrofti* are similar. However, the former parasite has a shorter developmental cycle in the mosquito. Microfilariae often appear sooner after infection with this helminth.

4. The diagnosis of lymphatic filariasis caused by *B. malayi* may be made by the microscopic observation of the characteristic microfilariae, having terminal and subterminal nuclei extending to the tips of the tails, in Giemsa- or hematoxylin-stained thick and thin blood smears. The Knott concentration technique or filtration of blood through a Nuclepore filter may be useful in light infections (for details of these techniques, see case 47).

   However, microfilariae are not always demonstrable in infected patients. In some cases, the worm burden is too light for detection. This is especially true in nonnative persons traveling to areas of endemic infection. For diagnosis of infection in these patients, a wide variety of serological methods are available. These procedures are of little value in native populations, since most of these individuals have a positive serological response. In many cases, the presence of the signs and symptoms of filariasis may be sufficient to make a presumptive diagnosis.

5. The usual treatment for filariasis is diethylcarbamazine or ivermectin. Lower doses of diethylcarbamazine are recommended for brugian filariasis, due to the frequency of severe reactions. Side effects are probably due to destruction of the microfilariae and adult worms and are not directly caused by the drug. This drug may be used in combination with albendazole and is especially useful in India, where ivermectin may not be readily available.

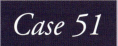

Case 51

A 59-year-old woman whose husband raised pigs for home use was seen by her family practitioner with symptoms of fever, weakness, severe muscle pain and joint aches, which she described as "flu-like" symptoms. She had suffered from diarrhea, nausea, and abdominal cramps a month or two earlier. On physical examination, the patient was noted to have periorbital edema. Based on this finding, the examining physician asked about her food habits. She admitted to a fondness for eating homemade pork sausage.

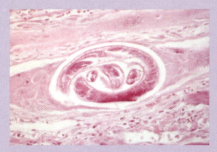

Laboratory blood tests revealed eosinophilia (50%). A muscle biopsy specimen was taken from her biceps muscle, and an encysted helminth larva was identified (Fig. 51.1). An inflammatory infiltrate was also noted.

Figure 51.1

QUESTIONS

1. Which infection does this patient have?

2. How is this infection transmitted? Which factor in the patient's history put her at risk of this infection?

3. Describe the life cycle of this helminth.

4. Correlate this patient's symptoms with the life cycle of this nematode. Which other conditions may be confused with this infection?

5. How does infection with this nematode differ from many other helminthic infections?

6. In which type of muscle is this parasite most likely to be found? How is the muscle tissue examined?

7. In addition to eosinophilia and muscle biopsy findings, which other abnormal laboratory results are common in this infection?

8. How is this infection prevented?

9. How is this infection treated?

ANSWERS

1. This patient has trichinosis (trichinellosis) caused by the nematode *Trichinella spiralis*, which is distributed worldwide. There are actually five or six known species of *Trichinella*. All species are morphologically similar, and any of the species may cause trichinosis. However, in the United States, only *T. spiralis* is usually seen. In this case, *T. spiralis* was identified by DNA analysis.

2. Human infection with *T. spiralis* results from the ingestion of poorly cooked meat, usually pork but also meat from bears, walruses, horses, or other mammals (carnivores and omnivores) infected with viable, infective larvae. Most cases of trichinosis in the United States are derived from home-raised rather than commercially raised pigs. The fact that this patient was fond of eating homemade pork sausage made from home-raised pigs put her at risk of contracting trichinosis.

Trichinosis may also be acquired from eating game meat. Hunters are known to cook bear meat as they would beef steaks. Inadequately cooked bear meat is a frequent source of infection with *T. spiralis*.

3. First-stage larvae of *T. spiralis* which have been ingested in infected meat and which are resistant to gastric juices are released from digested meat in the stomach. Larvae penetrate the intestinal wall, develop through four larval stages, mature, and mate in the upper intestine by the second day. Larvae may be produced within 3 days of fertilization. The duration of the intestinal phase varies depending on the worm burden and the immune status of the host.

Motile larvae are carried by the intestinal lymphatics or mesenteric venules to body tissues, particularly to striated muscle tissue. The larvae penetrate the sheaths of the muscle fibers. They coil in spirals in muscle tissue and become encysted within a few weeks. Encysted larvae may remain viable for many years, although calcification may occur within a year.

4. Trichinosis may be divided into three phases: the intestinal phase, the muscle invasion phase, and the convalescent phase. Symptoms in any phase of infection are usually based on the number of ingested cysts. Other factors influencing the disease are the patient's age, size, and general health.

The previous symptoms of diarrhea, nausea, and abdominal cramps reported by this patient were typical of the intestinal phase of infection. These symptoms may occur within 24 h of ingestion and may suggest food poisoning. Diarrhea may last up to 14 weeks, with no muscle invasion. During the muscle invasion phase, fever, facial (especially periorbital) edema, weakness and muscle pain may develop. Muscle damage may cause difficulty in swallowing, breathing, etc., depending on the muscles involved. Myocarditis may develop after the third week. Death may occur between the fourth and eighth weeks. Central nervous system involvement, although rare, is life-threatening. During the convalescent phase, usually after several months, worms die, and cyst calcification occurs.

Mild cases of trichinosis with a low loading dose may cause flu-like symptoms. Other diagnoses which might be considered include bacterial food poisoning and typhoid fever.

5. Unlike many helminths, all stages of development (adult and larva) of *T. spiralis* occur in a single host. There is no egg stage in the life cycle of this nematode.

6. Encysted larvae of *T. spiralis* are most likely to be observed in very active muscle tissue having the greatest blood supply, such as the diaphragm and muscles of the larynx, neck, jaws, tongue, ribs, biceps, and gastrocnemius. Muscle tissue obtained at biopsy may be examined by compressing the tissue between two glass slides and observing the preparation microscopically using the low-power (10×) objective. Alternatively, muscle tissue may be examined by using an artificial digestion method to release larvae from the specimen. Infected meat may also be examined in this manner.

7. In addition to eosinophilia and abnormal histological results, other abnormal laboratory findings in patients with trichinosis include elevated levels of serum muscle enzymes, including lactic dehydrogenase, aldolase, creatinine phosphokinase, and aspartate aminotransferase, and abnormally high immunoglobulin E levels. Serological tests, including an enzyme immunoassay and the bentonite flocculation test, may be useful in the diagnosis of this infection.

8. Trichinosis may be prevented by proper cooking of meats, especially pork, although outbreaks have been reported due to consumption of improperly cooked horsemeat. Storage of meats at low temperatures (−15°C for 20 days or more) decreases the viability of the parasite. Freezing or the use of a microwave oven does not necessarily kill all larvae of this parasite.

Although laws exist banning the feeding of uncooked garbage to pigs commercially, these regulations do not apply to home use. Educational efforts should be made to discourage farmers from feeding slaughterhouse scraps and uncooked garbage containing pork scraps to hogs raised for home use.

9. Treatment depends on the phase of infection. During the early stage, the goal is to minimize the number of larvae. During the intestinal phase, mebendazole or albendazole is recommended. For treatment of severe infection, steroids may be added. Supportive therapy may be the only option during the muscle invasion phase.

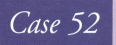

Case 52

An 18-year-old male migrant worker from Mexico presented to an emergency department in California complaining of visual disturbances and blurred vision. He also complained of itching that was so severe that he had been unable to sleep. Physical examination revealed dermatitis and several painless nodules on his scalp. Eye examination revealed tiny ophthalmic lesions on his right cornea.

Based on the patient's nodules, his previous residence in Mexico, and his ocular involvement, the physician suspected that he had a condition known as river blindness. A tiny bit of skin was taken for examination. A wet preparation in saline was viewed microscopically. Unsheathed microfilariae with tapered tails were observed microscopically. A microfilaria is shown in Fig. 52.1.

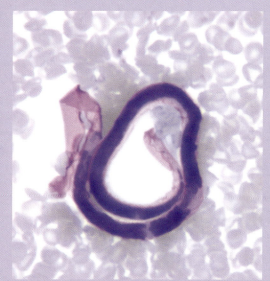

Figure 52.1

QUESTIONS

1. Which infection does this patient have?

2. Why is this infection referred to as river blindness?

3. What is the name given to the nodules found on this patient's scalp?

4. What is the intermediate host for this parasite?

5. Describe the life cycle of this parasite.

6. How is the diagnosis of this infection made?

7. How is this infection treated?

ANSWERS

1. This patient has onchocerciasis caused by the filarial nematode *Onchocerca volvulus*.

2. This infection is commonly called river blindness because ocular lesions often seen in patients with onchocerciasis may progress to blindness and because the habitats of the insect vectors are rivers and streams. The degree of eye involvement is related to the duration and severity of infection.

This infection is a widespread cause of blindness in Africa, Mexico, and parts of Central and South America. Its distribution is limited to areas hospitable to its vectors and in close proximity to rivers or streams, where larvae and pupae develop. Surgical removal of the nodules, especially those on the scalp, has been shown to markedly decrease the ocular complications of onchocerciasis.

3. The painless subcutaneous nodules found on this patient's scalp, which are characteristic of this infection and which contain adult worms, are known as onchocercomas. Although these nodules may be found on the trunk or limbs of patients in Africa and Venezuela, they are frequently found on the scalp of patients in Mexico and Guatemala.

4. The intermediate host for *O. volvulus* is the blackfly or gnat in the genus *Simulium*.

5. The blackfly or gnat ingests microfilariae from an infected person. Microfilariae develop into infective larvae, which migrate to the mouthparts of the intermediate host. Humans are infected as the fly takes another blood meal, when infective larvae are deposited on the skin and enter the bite wound. The developing worms migrate through subcutaneous and connective tissues in the human host. Most worms become encapsulated, forming nodules. Adult worms produce unsheathed microfilariae, which invade the subcutaneous tissues, the skin, and the eyes.

6. The diagnosis of onchocerciasis is made be detecting the unsheathed microfilariae, which have body nuclei that do not extend to the tip of the tail, in "skin snips." These bits of tissue may be sliced thinly with a corneal-scleral punch, scalpel, or razor blade. The specimen is incubated for 30 min to 2 h in saline to allow migration of microfilariae from the tissue to the liquid phase. Multiple skin snips should be examined in cases of light infection.

7. Surgical removal of nodules is usually indicated. This is true especially for nodules on the head, to reduce ocular complications. Regional lymph glands may also be removed. Ivermectin is the drug of choice for treating onchocerciasis. This drug greatly reduces the microfilarial burden of the host and decreases the prevalence of ocular microfilariae, with improved visual acuity. Diethylcarbamazine is an effective drug but has more serious side effects. Other agents include suramin, amocarzine, mebendazole, and flubendazole.

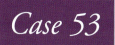

Case 53

A 2-year-old girl was brought to the emergency department suffering from signs of meningoencephalitis. She lived in a rural, wooded area in California and had no history of travel. Cerebrospinal fluid specimens were negative for bacterial and viral pathogens. Blood tests revealed eosinophilia (40%). She was admitted to the intensive care unit, where she remained for 5 weeks. During this time, her condition deteriorated and she died on the 40th hospital day.

On autopsy, many granulomas containing nematode larvae were seen in several organs and tissues, including the brain. The patient was diagnosed with eosinophilic meningoencephalitis.

QUESTIONS

1. Which nematode caused this patient's infection?

2. How is this infection transmitted to humans?

3. Describe the life cycle of this nematode.

4. Discuss the symptoms of this disease.

5. How is the diagnosis of this infection made?

6. How can this infection be prevented?

7. Is there an effective treatment for this infection?

ANSWERS

1. This patient is infected with the nematode *Baylisascaris procyonis,* an ascarid found in raccoons.

2. This infection is acquired by humans, usually young children, by the fecal-oral route, when eggs of *B. procyonis* are accidentally ingested. These eggs are passed in very large numbers in the feces of infected raccoons. The eggs are sticky, which makes them difficult to remove from hands or toys. Although the eggs need to develop for 2 to 3 weeks before becoming infective, infants commonly put many things in their mouths and are therefore more likely to become exposed to the eggs of *B. procyonis.*

Raccoons tend to defecate in common areas called latrines. Latrines may be located on the ground, on roofs, and in attics. The eggs remain viable for extended periods, perhaps years.

3. Raccoons become infected with *B. procyonis* by ingesting infective eggs or by ingesting larvae encapsulated in the tissues of rodents or other animals. In the raccoon, larvae hatch and enter the wall of the small intestine, where they develop to maturity. Infected raccoons shed large numbers of eggs in their feces.

After ingestion by humans or a number of other birds and mammals, the ascarid eggs hatch in the intestinal tract, releasing immature larvae. The larvae do not develop to adult worms, as they do in the raccoon. Instead, they migrate through tissues. This extraintestinal migration is called larva migrans and may affect the viscera, causing visceral larva migrans (VLM), resulting in tissue inflammation; the eyes, causing ocular larva migrans (OLM); or the central nervous system, causing neural larva migrans (NLM). OLM frequently accompanies NLM in children. OLM results in a unilateral neuroretinitis in adults. Larval migration may result in permanent neurological damage, blindness, or death.

4. Symptoms of infection with *B. procyonis* include eosinophilic meningoencephalitis or unilateral neuroretinitis, depending on the number of eggs ingested. OLM may be accompanied by chronic endophthalmitis with retinal detachment, keratitis, uveitis, iritis, and posterior-pole granuloma. NLM may be accompanied by symptoms ranging from mild neuropsychological problems to seizures, convulsions, and ataxia. Patients may suddenly become lethargic or irritable and may lose muscle coordination and head control. Spasmodic contractions of neck muscles, stupor, coma, and death may follow.

5. Human infections with *B. procyonis* are rare and difficult to diagnose and may be recognized only by a process of elimination of other causes of larva migrans. The disease is probably underrecognized, and the full spectrum of illness has not been defined. There have been 11 documented cases, all but 1 (in a 17-year-old male) occurring in young children. Results of routine hematological and cerebrospinal fluid studies are usually consistent with a parasitic infection but are nonspecific.

The definitive diagnosis of bayliascariasis is usually made by the morphological identification of the larvae of *B. procyonis* in tissue. These larvae, although generally larger than others, must be morphologically distinguished from those of *Toxo-*

cara canis, *T. cati, Ascaris lumbricoides*, and species of *Gnathastoma, Angio-strongylus*, and *Ancylostoma*, as well as several cestode larvae causing cysticercosis and echinococcosis.

If this infection is misdiagnosed, extensive damage is likely to occur, with devastating consequences.

6. Baylisascariasis is a serious emerging helminthic zoonotic infection with the potential to cause serious illness and death, especially in young children. Successful control of this infection requires efforts to prevent the establishment of raccoon latrine sites in areas where humans live and are likely to come in contact. Educational efforts should stress the importance of not feeding raccoons or keeping them as pets. Food sources should be protected from raccoon access.

7. There is no effective cure for baylisascariasis. Steroids may be used to treat symptoms. Anthelmintics such as albendazole and ivermectin are usually not effective in treating NLM. Ocular infections may be treated by laser photocoagulation therapy to kill the intraretinal larvae.

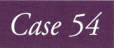

Case 54   A previously healthy 28-year-old man presented to the emergency department of a hospital in downtown San Francisco with severe abdominal pain, nausea, and vomiting. He had had dinner a few days earlier in a local Asian restaurant, where he had eaten sushi.

Due to his severe pain, a gastroscopic examination was performed. Nematode larvae were visualized and removed. The patient's symptoms subsided shortly thereafter.

QUESTIONS

1. Which nematode is likely to be responsible for this patient's symptoms?

2. What aspect of the patient's history would make you suspect this infection?

3. Describe the life cycle of this nematode.

4. Discuss the symptoms of this infection.

5. How is the diagnosis of this infection made?

6. What is the treatment of choice for this infection?

ANSWERS

1. The likely helminth responsible for this patient's symptoms is *Anisakis simplex*. Other nematodes in the family Anisakidae which may cause this syndrome include species of *Pseudoterranova,* which is actually a more common cause of anisakiasis in the United States.

2. Anisakiasis is acquired by the ingestion of raw, pickled, salted, smoked, or insufficiently cooked saltwater fish or squid. The patient reported that he had had dinner several days earlier in a restaurant where he ordered a meal (sushi), which must have included infected fish.

3. The primary hosts of *Anisakis* are marine mammals, including dolphins, porpoises, seals, sea lions, and whales. These mammals ingest third-stage larvae, which embed in clusters in the stomach wall and develop into mature worms. Eggs produced by the female worms are passed out into the sea in feces of the mammal.

   The eggs become embryonated in the sea water. First-stage larvae develop, which molt into second-stage larvae. Second-stage larvae are hatched from the eggs and are ingested by tiny marine crustaceans. In the crustaceans, second-stage larvae develop into third-stage larvae. These larvae are infective for fish and squid and may be passed from fish to fish, where they may be found in viscera or muscle. Fish at the top of the food chain may become heavily infected. Fish and squid contain third-stage larvae, which are infective for sea mammals and humans. If ingested by sea mammals, the larvae develop into adult worms, thus completing the life cycle. If consumed by humans, the larvae are unable to complete the life cycle.

4. In humans, larvae often penetrate the wall of the digestive tract, usually the stomach but also the intestine. Symptoms of nausea and vomiting may begin in about 24 h. After penetration, they may become embedded in eosinophilic granulomas. Symptoms of anisakiasis may be evident in several hours after ingestion of infected fish or squid but are more common after 1 to 5 days.

   It is known that *A. simplex* can cause allergic reactions in sensitized individuals. These reactions generally occur only when the parasites are viable and infective. There have been two reported cases of pulmonary anisakiasis in humans. These cases were also associated with the consumption of raw fish.

5. Diagnosis of anisakiasis may be made by gastroscopic examination, during which the larvae may be visualized. Larvae are sometimes vomited by the patient. They may also be seen during histopathological examination of granulomatous tissue taken from the intestine during biopsy. A history of eating fish within the past few days is helpful in making the diagnosis.

6. No treatment is needed for transient anisakiasis. The treatment of choice for gastrointestinal anisakiasis when worms are embedded in the stomach or bowel wall is surgical or endoscopic removal of the larvae. Third-stage larvae measure 1 to 3 cm (or more) long by 1 cm wide. Albendazole is recommended as supplementary therapy.

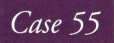

Case 55

The patient was a 3-year-old girl who was seen by her pediatrician for a routine physical examination. Her mother was concerned about her daughter's poor appetite. Physical examination revealed that the child was small for her age and had a slightly enlarged liver. Blood was collected for a routine complete blood count, since she had previously been slightly anemic. Her hemoglobin level was within the normal range; however, she did have eosinophilia (20%).

The child had no history of travel. When questioned about pets, her mother reported that she spent a great deal of time with her puppy. Suspicion of a helminthic infection caused the physician to send blood to a state reference laboratory, where a serological procedure was performed to confirm the diagnosis.

QUESTIONS

1. Which parasitic infection might be responsible for this patient's symptoms?

2. What is the significance of the child having a puppy?

3. How is this infection acquired?

4. Describe the life cycle of this parasite.

5. Which two manifestations of this infection are known to occur?

6. How is this infection usually diagnosed?

7. How is this infection usually treated?

8. How can this infection be prevented?

ANSWERS

1. This patient has VLM, a zoonotic infection caused by the nematode *Toxocara canis,* a dog parasite, or the cat ascarid *Toxocara cati,* among others. Since the child had a puppy, her infection was probably due to infection with the former helminth.

2. The highest rates of *T. canis* infections have been found in puppies, which acquire infection from their mothers transplacentally or through the mother's milk. Puppies may begin shedding eggs at 2 weeks of age, and most of them recover from the infection in 3 to 6 months. A small number of dogs continue to host patent infections past 6 months of age, and these infections probably persist for life. Eggs become infective in about 3 weeks and remain viable in the soil for months.

At about 6 months of age, the immune system of the puppy has matured and become sufficiently competent to result in passage of the worms from the intestine. After this time, any infectious larvae ingested migrate out of the gut and encyst in various places in the body. In an immunocompetent male dog, these larvae remain in the encysted stage until the death of the dog. In a female dog, reactivation of the encysted larvae (or a number of them) occurs during pregnancy. The larvae pass into the bloodstream, migrate across the placenta, and infect the pups in utero. If dogs have a compromised immune system, it is possible that encysted *T. canis* larvae could become reactivated and cause a patent infection.

Approximately 50% of puppies and 20% of mature dogs harbor this parasite. The older animals probably acquire the infection by the ingestion of infective eggs from the soil or in infected rats or mice. When the infected rodents are eaten, the larvae complete their development in the dog's intestine.

3. This infection is acquired by humans by the accidental ingestion of infective eggs of *T. canis* or *T. cati* in contaminated soil. A case of toxocariasis in an adult, based on serological findings, has been reported to be caused by the ingestion of raw lamb liver.

4. Nematode eggs are shed in the feces of dogs and cats. The eggs mature in the soil and become infective in 2 or 3 weeks. After ingestion by a human, usually a young child, the larvae hatch in the small intestine and penetrate the intestinal wall. Larvae do not develop to adulthood as they do in dogs; instead, they migrate to the liver. Larvae may migrate to the lungs or to other parts of the body including the brain, heart, muscle, and eyes, or they may remain in the liver. They may become encapsulated in dense fibrous tissue. Larvae do not mature, even if they migrate back to the intestine.

5. This nematode may cause VLM or, rarely, OLM. In the latter condition, a granulomatous reaction may occur in the retina. OLM tends to occur in older children, while VLM occurs mostly in younger children. OLM may be confused with retinoblastoma, ocular tumors, and other childhood eye problems. VLM symptoms caused by *T. canis* must be differentiated from those caused by other helminths which migrate through tissue.

This infection usually does not cause serious problems. Many patients, like the patient described in this case, are asymptomatic but have a high rate of eosinophilia. Many of these cases go unrecognized.

6. Although the diagnosis of toxocariasis may be confirmed by the identification of nematode larvae in biopsy specimens, this approach is not recommended. Serological assays are available through state departments of health, which often forward these specimens to the Centers for Disease Control and Prevention for testing.

7. The disease may be self-limited. Some cases of toxocariasis respond to treatment with diethylcarbamizine, thiabendazole, ivermectin, or albendazole. In cases of OLM, larvae in the eye may be destroyed by photocoagulation. Steroids may be included in the treatment of severe cases of OLM and VLM. Treatment is facilitated by a prompt diagnosis.

8. Dogs should be seen regularly by a veterinarian for deworming. Children should not be allowed to eat dirt. Dogs should be leashed and prevented from defecating in public places, such as parks.

   Toxocara eggs have been found in many soil specimens collected from both public parks and private yards and gardens. Sandboxes in public parks, as well in private yards, should be protected from contamination by these eggs. This can be accomplished by covering them with clear vinyl sheets at night and during rainy weather.

REFERENCES

Cairncross, S. C., R. Muller, and N. Zagaria. 2002. Dracunculiasis (guinea worm disease) and the eradication initiative. *Clin. Microbiol. Rev.* **15:**223–246.

Centers for Disease Control and Prevention. 2003. Progress toward global eradication of dracunuliasis, January–June 2003. *Morb. Mortal. Wkly. Rep.* **52:**881–883.

Garcia, L. S. 2001. *Diagnostic Medical Parasitology,* 4th ed. ASM Press, Washington, D.C.

Heelan, J. S., and F. W. Ingersoll. 2002. *Essentials of Human Parasitology.* Thomson Delmar Learning, Albany, N.Y.

Markell, E. K., D. T. John, and W. A. Krotoski. 1999. *Markell and Voge's Medical Parasitology,* 8th ed., p. 304–356. The W. B. Saunders Co., Philadelphia, Pa.

Salem, G., and P. Schantz. 1992. Toxocaral visceral larva migrans after ingestion of raw lamb liver. *Clin. Infect. Dis.* **15:**743–744.

Sorvillo, F., L. R. Ash, O. G. W. Berlin, J. Yatabe, C. Degiorgio, and S. A. Morse. 2002. *Baylisascaris procyonis:* an emerging helminthic zoonosis. *Emerg. Infect. Dis.* **8:**355–359.

Zeibig, E. A. 1997. *Clinical Parasitology.* The W. B. Saunders Co., Philadelphia, Pa.

This section includes cases in which patients present to their physicians or to the emergency department with gastrointestinal symptoms, such as diarrhea, nausea, and abdominal pain, which might suggest an infection with intestinal parasites. Bacteria and viruses may also cause gastrointestinal symptoms and must be considered in the differential diagnosis. Noninfectious causes of these symptoms must also be considered. The reader must develop a differential diagnosis to exclude (or identify) parasites as potential infectious agents, which may be a challenge; hence the title of this section.

The reader may refer to Section I for information on nonpathogenic intestinal protozoa, which might be present in healthy individuals. It might be tempting to "blame" these innocent bystanders for the patient's symptoms. The danger in making this diagnosis would be to overlook the true cause of the patient's symptoms, which might put the patient at risk. The patient might also receive inappropriate therapy to treat harmless microorganisms.

Routine stool cultures detect the most common bacteria which cause gastrointestinal infections; these include *Salmonella* species, *Shigella* species, and *Campylobacter jejuni*. Cultures for the enteric pathogens *Yersinia enterocolitica* and *Vibrio* species, which require special media, are usually available on request. Diarrheagenic *Escherichia coli* may be cultured routinely or only on request. Infection with *Clostridium difficile* may also cause gastrointestinal symptoms.

Viruses which may cause gastrointestinal symptoms include rotaviruses, enteric adenoviruses, astroviruses, and noroviruses.

Noninfectious causes of diarrhea and other gastrointestinal symptoms include inflammatory bowel disease such as ulcerative colitis, with symptoms closely resembling those of amebiasis, and Crohn's disease.

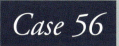

Case 56

A 35-year-old woman presented to her primary-care doctor with gastrointestinal symptoms including diarrhea, abdominal pain, and nausea of several weeks' duration. The patient's travel history was unremarkable. However, she noted that a day before her symptoms began, she had eaten chicken still "pink" inside. The patient's physician ordered a stool specimen for culture for *Salmonella* and *Shigella* and three specimens for routine examination for ova and parasites.

Cultures were reported to be "negative for *Salmonella* and *Shigella*." No parasites were seen in the sediments prepared from the concentrated specimens. Two of the three permanent stained trichrome smears were reported negative, but the third specimen showed a few pear-shaped trophozoites, measuring 6 to 16 μm by 6 to 9 μm. A single nucleus, containing a small, central karyosome, was present in the anterior part of the trophozoite. Each trophozoite was characterized by the presence of an undulating membrane which extended for the length of the cell. A central, longitudinal axostyle, which curved around the nucleus and extended posteriorly beyond the cell, was present in each trophozoite. No peripheral chromatin was observed in the nucleus.

QUESTIONS

1. Which intestinal parasite would fit the description given?

2. Is this parasite considered to be a pathogen? If not, which bacterial agent might be causing this patient's symptoms?

3. How would the presence of this pathogen correlate with the patient's history?

4. Which laboratory test could help this physician make a diagnosis of this infection?

5. Why is the new name appropriate for this parasite?

6. What is the function of the axostyle?

7. Why were no cysts seen in any of the microscopic preparations?

8. How is this parasite detected?

9. How is this parasite transmitted? How can infection with this parasite be prevented?

ANSWERS

1. The morphology of the trophozoites in the permanent smear would fit the description of the intestinal protozoan *Pentatrichomonas (Trichomonas) hominis*.

2. No. *P. hominis* is a nonpathogen. In this case, bacterial cultures were able to rule out *Salmonella* and *Shigella*; however, no culture was done to detect the commonly isolated enteric pathogen *Campylobacter jejuni*.

3. The patient had reportedly eaten "pink" or undercooked chicken. *C. jejuni* is known to be associated with poultry, and infection with this pathogen is often transmitted by the ingestion of undercooked poultry or poorly cooked food (such as rare hamburger) that has been contaminated by infected poultry.

4. Although most laboratories look for *Salmonella*, *Shigella*, and *Campylobacter* species in routine stool cultures, this laboratory reported only "negative for *Salmonella* and *Shigella*." Therefore, a stool specimen should be submitted for culture for *C. jejuni*. Most laboratories include this pathogen when a routine stool culture is ordered. A selective medium for the isolation of *C. jejuni* should be inoculated and incubated in a microaerophilic atmosphere for cultivation of this organism. Many laboratories grow this organism in 48 h at 42°C in this atmosphere.

5. The "penta" refers to the five anterior flagella found on *P. hominis*. Although not usually seen microscopically, four of these flagella arise anteriorly; the fifth flagellum also arises anteriorly and then runs to the posterior end of the cell, forming the outer edge of the undulating membrane. It extends behind the trophozoite as a free flagellum.

6. The axostyle of *P. hominis* runs through the cell from the anterior to the posterior end and extends beyond the posterior end. This sharply pointed structure provides rigidity to the cell.

7. *P. hominis* is not known to have a cyst form.

8. Although the trophozoites of this flagellate are small, they may be seen moving in saline wet mounts of diarrheic stools. The flagella and the undulating membrane often do not stain well with the permanent stain and might not be easily visualized. However, the nucleus at the anterior end of the trophozoite and the costa are more likely to be visible. These structures and cytoplasmic granules are diagnostic for this parasite. The trichrome stain is preferred over the iron hematoxylin stain to make this diagnosis.

9. Infection with *P. hominis* occurs worldwide but is especially common in children living in warm climates. It is thought that the trophozoite form may be transmitted in a material such as milk, which would protect the trophozites from destruction in the stomach. This protection allows the organism to reach the intestine.

    P. hominis infection may be prevented by improving personal hygiene practices and sanitary methods to reduce fecal-oral transmission.

A 36-year-old man who had recently returned from a camping trip presented to the emergency department with complaints of nausea, diarrhea, and vomiting of several days' duration. His physical examination was unremarkable.

A stool specimen was collected and submitted for routine bacterial culture and examination for ova and parasites. The specimen was a liquid stool sample delivered to the laboratory and examined immediately. Trophozoites exhibiting sluggish, nonprogressive motility were seen on examination of the saline wet mount. A small number of ameboid trophozoites, measuring 8 to 20 μm, with coarsely granular cytoplasm and no peripheral nuclear chromatin, were seen in the permanent trichrome stain. No ingested red blood cells were visible. A large karyosome filled much of the intranuclear space. A characteristic trophozoite is shown in Fig. 57.1. No cyst forms were seen. The results of the stool culture were not yet available.

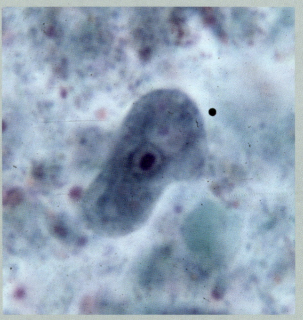

Figure 57.1

QUESTIONS

1. Based on the figure shown, which parasite would you identify?

2. Should this patient be treated? Why or why not?

3. Describe the life cycle of this parasite.

4. Which other frequently encountered intestinal amebae may be confused with this parasite? How would you morphologically differentiate these protozoans from each other?

5. Which other infectious agents might be causing this patient's symptoms?

ANSWERS

1. Based on the description of the trophozoites of this parasite, we can conclude that this parasite is the ameba *Iodamoeba bütschlii*. Apparently there were no cysts present; this is to be expected in a diarrheal specimen, which is likely to contain only trophozoites. The trophozoite of this parasite lacks peripheral nuclear chromatin and is characterized by the presence of a large, blotlike karyosome. The cyst form of *I. bütschlii* contains a large glycogen vacuole, which stains reddish brown with iodine and appears as a clear unstained space when observed in the trichrome permanent stain.

2. The patient should not be treated for his parasitic infection. *I. bütschlii* is non-pathogenic and has not been associated with human disease. The pathogenic ameba *Entamoeba histolytica*, if present, should be treated with metronidazole or another amebicidal agent such as iodoquinol or diloxanide furoate. The results of the stool culture might indicate treatment of this patient with antibiotics.

3. Infection with *I. bütschlii* begins when mature cysts (the infective stage) are ingested. The mature cyst passes through the stomach and excysts in the lower ileum of the small intestine. Here the cyst develops into the trophozoite form and multiplies by binary fission. Trophozoites continue to multiply in the lumen of the colon. They may encyst and pass from the body in the feces.

4. Other frequently encountered intestinal amebae which must be distinguished from *I. bütschlii* include *E. histolytica*, *E. dispar*, *Endolimax nana*, *E. hartmanni*, and *Entamoeba coli*.

Direct saline wet preparations may be useful in detecting motile trophozoites, especially in liquid stool specimens, although most fecal specimens for ova and parasites are collected in preservatives. Concentration techniques may allow the observation of amebic cysts. However, a permanent smear, stained with the trichrome or iron hematoxylin stain, is most useful in the identification of amebic trophozoites and cysts. A permanent stained smear should be made with all stool specimens, regardless of the consistency of the specimen. A minimum of three specimens should be collected over 10 days.

E. histolytica is the only pathogen among this group of parasites. The trophozoites of this protozoan measure 12 to 60 μm, have finely granular cytoplasm and evenly distributed peripheral nuclear chromatin, and frequently reveal ingested red blood cells. Cyst forms measure 10 to 20 μm and contain four nuclei plus cigar-shaped chromatoid bodies with smooth, rounded, blunt ends. Although immature cysts (with one or two nuclei) may be passed in the feces, cysts may develop to maturity (with four nuclei) before being excreted. Trophozoites, immature cysts, and mature cysts may be found in the feces, although trophozoites are usually found only in liquid feces. *E. dispar* is morphologically indistinguishable from *E. histolytica*; however, red blood cells are not ingested.

E. hartmanni is morphologically similar to *E. histolytica* but is smaller. The ameboid trophozoites of this parasite measure 5 to 12 μm, with finely granular cytoplasm and evenly distributed peripheral nuclear chromatin. No ingested red blood cells are seen. Cyst forms measure 5 to 10 μm, and each contains two to four nuclei and cigar-shaped chromatoid bodies (chromatoid bars) with smooth, rounded, blunt ends.

The trophozoite of *Entamoeba coli* measures 15 to 50 μm. The coarsely granulated cytoplasm of this parasite is often described as "dirty," due to the presence of many vacuoles plus bacteria, yeasts, and debris. Peripheral nuclear chromatin is present in the nucleus and is unevenly distributed in clumps. The nucleus contains a large, discrete eccentric karyosome. The characteristic motility of *Entamoeba coli* has been described as sluggish and nonprogressive. The cyst is spherical or oval, measures 10 to 35 μm, and contains 8 (sometimes 16) nuclei when mature; immature cysts contain fewer than 8 nuclei. Peripheral chromatin is present and is granular and unevenly distributed. Chromatoidal bars have sharp, pointed ends.

Endolimax nana is morphologically most similar to and thus most likely to be confused with *I. bütschlii*. The trophozoite of *Endolimax nana* measures 6 to 12 μm, has finely vacuolated cytoplasm, and lacks peripheral nuclear chromatin. Usually, only a large, blotlike karyosome is visible in the nucleus. The cysts of *Endolimax nana* contain four nuclei, lack chromatoid bodies, and measure 5 to 10 μm.

5. The patient might be infected with pathogenic bacilli, such as *Shigella, Salmonella,* or *Campylobacter* species. These enteric bacilli may be isolated when a routine bacterial culture of a stool specimen is ordered. Cultures for *Yersinia* and *Vibrio* species, which are also enteric pathogens, are usually performed on request, based on clinical findings. Treatment with antimicrobial agents might be indicated based on culture results.

Infection with *Clostridium difficile* (not likely in this patient) also causes diarrhea in patients who have received long-course antibiotic treatment. The patient might be suffering from antibiotic-associated diarrhea or the more serious pseudomembranous colitis caused by this anaerobic bacterium. This bacterium is not usually identified when a routine culture for enteric pathogens is ordered. Rapid enzyme immunoassays and tissue culture methods are commercially available for the detection of toxins produced by *C. difficile.*

Viruses such as noroviruses may also cause similar symptoms. These viruses are especially common in settings of crowding and inadequate sanitation and have caused camping-related outbreaks. Viral cultures and/or enzyme immunoassays for these viruses and other selected agents are generally available.

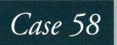

Case 58

A 28-year-old man visited his family doctor complaining of crampy abdominal pain, malaise, nausea, fever, and bloody diarrhea. He had been passing 8 to 10 loose stools daily for several weeks. Stool specimens were collected on three alternate days and sent to the laboratory for routine examination for ova and parasites; one specimen was submitted for routine bacterial culture.

The stool culture was negative for bacterial pathogens. Although no parasites were recognizable in the concentrated sediments of the specimens, a small number of ameboid trophozoites, measuring 20 to 30 μm, with finely granular cytoplasm and evenly distributed peripheral nuclear chromatin, were seen in the permanent trichrome stains of two of the three specimens. No ingested red blood cells were visible. A characteristic trophozoite is shown in Fig. 58.1. No cyst forms were seen. A report of "*Entamoeba histolytica* present" was sent to the ordering physician by the laboratory.

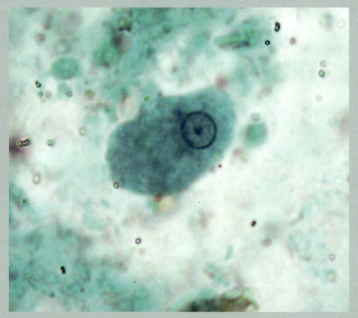

Figure 58.1

To confirm the diagnosis of amebic dysentery, the patient's physician ordered an immunoassay for *E. histolytica* on a fresh stool specimen. The immunoassay was able to rule out infection with *E. histolytica*. A report of "no *Entamoeba histolytica* antigen detected" was received by the physician. When the patient's symptoms continued, a colonoscopy was performed and a diagnosis of ulcerative colitis was made.

QUESTIONS

1. How would you explain the discrepancy between the microscopic examination and the immunoassay results?

2. How should the results of the ova and parasite examination have been reported?

3. How do the symptoms of amebic dysentery mimic those of ulcerative colitis?

4. Describe the advantages and disadvantages of the immunoassays used to test for *E. histolytica* and *E. dispar?*

5. Describe the life cycles of these two parasites. How do they differ?

6. Describe the ulcers formed in severe cases of amebic dysentery.

ANSWERS

1. The description of the parasites seen in the permanent smear closely resembles the description of the pathogenic *E. histolytica.* The trophozoites of this parasite measure 12 to 60 μm, with finely granular cytoplasm and evenly distributed peripheral nuclear chromatin. The patient's symptoms of bloody diarrhea, abdominal pain, nausea, fever, and malaise also support the diagnosis of amebiasis or amebic dysentery.

The nonpathogenic *E. dispar* is morphologically indistinguishable from *E. histolytica.* *E. histolytica* and *E. dispar* are now considered to be two separate species. The only morphological characteristic that may be used to differentiate the two parasites is the ingestion of red blood cells characteristic of *E. histolytica,* although it is not uncommon to see trophozoites without red blood cells in the cytoplasm, even in cases of bloody diarrhea. Red blood cells are not found in the trophozoites of *E. dispar.*

The trophozoites seen in the trichrome-stained smears were those of *E. dispar.* This was a coincidental finding and was unrelated to the patient's symptoms. The immunoassay was specific for the diagnosis of *E. histolytica* and was negative for this pathogen. The patient's symptoms were due to his ulcerative colitis.

2. The protozoan parasites seen microscopically in the permanent trichrome-stained smears should have been reported as members of the *E. histolytica/E. dispar* group.

3. The symptoms of ulcerative colitis closely resemble those of amebiasis and include frequent bowel movements with blood in the feces and crampy abdominal pain. In severe cases of inflammatory bowel disease (which includes ulcerative colitis and Crohn's disease), fever, anemia, and weight loss may also occur.

4. Although several immunoassays are available to detect the *E. histolytica/E. dispar* group, most fecal immunoassays are unable to distinguish between these two species. The advantage of the immunoassay used on this patient's specimen is its ability to make this distinction. However, these assays have limited use, since fresh or frozen stool is required but most fecal specimens are sent to the laboratory in vials of preservatives such as polyvinyl alcohol and formalin. The specimen submitted for this immunoassay was a fresh specimen and therefore was acceptable for testing.

5. The life cycles of the two amebae are similar. The infection begins when mature cysts (the infective stage) of *E. histolytica* or *E. dispar* are ingested. The mature cyst passes through the stomach and excysts in the lower ileum of the small intestine. Here the cyst develops into the trophozoite form and multiplies by binary fission. Trophozoites continue to multiply in the lumen of the colon, where they may encyst. Immature cysts (with one or two nuclei) are passed in the feces, although cysts may develop to maturity (with four nuclei) before being excreted. Trophozoites, immature cysts, and mature cysts may be found in the feces, although trophozoites are usually found only in liquid feces. Extraintestinal infection with *E. histolytica* occurs when amebic trophozoites invade the wall of the colon, enter the bloodstream, and spread to other areas of the body such as the lungs, spleen, and the brain, although liver abscesses are most common. Extraintestinal infection with *E. dispar* does not occur, because this species is nonpathogenic.

6. The "flask-shaped" ulcers characteristic of amebic dysentery have small openings on the mucosal surface, with a larger areas below the surface, giving the ulcers the flask shape. These ulcers often are found in the appendix, cecum, and ascending colon. The intestinal mucosa may appear normal between the ulcers.

Case 59

A previously healthy 56-year-old heterosexual man presented to his physician with complaints of bloody diarrhea, nausea, and abdominal pain. He had suffered these symptoms for about 1 week. He had no history of travel. His physician ordered three fecal specimens, collected on alternate days, to be sent to the laboratory for microscopic examination for ova and parasites, as well as a specimen for routine culture for enteric pathogens.

No parasites were seen in the wet mount from the concentrated sediment. However, a few teardrop-shaped protozoan trophozoites were seen in the permanent trichrome stains made from all three specimens. A prominent cytostome was visible in the trophozoite, extending approximately one-third of the length of the cell. A single nucleus was located in the anterior portion of the cell. These structures were identified as trophozoites of the flagellated protozoan *Chilomastix mesnili* (Fig. 59.1).

Two days later, along with members of the normal enteric bacterial flora, a lactose-negative gram-negative rod, identified as *Shigella dysenteriae*, was grown from the routine bacterial culture of the patient's stool specimen.

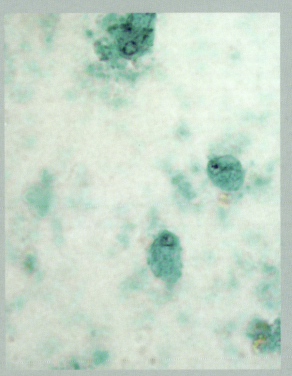

Figure 59.1

QUESTIONS

1. Which microorganism was most likely to be causing this patient's symptoms? Explain.

2. How are the trophozoites of the parasite shown in Fig. 59.1 distinguished morphologically from the pear-shaped trophozoites of the protozoan flagellate *Giardia lamblia*?

3. What is the significance to the clinician of the detection of *C. mesnili*?

4. Describe the appearance of the cyst stage of *C. mesnili*.

ANSWERS

1. The patient's symptoms were probably caused by infection with the bacterial pathogen *S. dysenteriae*. This bacterium causes bacillary dysentery, or shigellosis, with symptoms as described for this patient. The flagellated protozoan *C. mesnili* is not considered to be pathogenic in humans.

2. The trophozoite of *C. mesnili* slightly resembles that of *G. lamblia*, since they are both pear shaped. Although *C. mesnili* is generally smaller than *G. lamblia*, the ranges of sizes overlap. The trophozoite of *G. lamblia* is 9 to 20 μm long and 5 to 15 μm wide, while that of *C. mesnili* is 6 to 24 μm long by 5 to 8 μm wide.

   The trophozoite of *G. lamblia* has two nuclei, which are laterally located in the trophozoite. Each nucleus contains a large, central karyosome. An axostyle, consisting of two axonemes, divides the flagellate into symmetrical halves. Two curved median or parabasal bodies cross the axoneme at an oblique angle. Overall, these features give the trophozoite the appearance of a smiling face.

   The trophozoite of *C. mesnili* is elongated, pear shaped, or teardrop shaped, having a rounded anterior end which narrows to a pointed posterior end. A single large nucleus, which is located anteriorly at the rounded end of the trophozoite, has a small central or eccentric karyosome in the form of chromatin granules. No peripheral nuclear chromatin is present. A prominent cytostome, or oral groove, extends one-third to one-half of the length of the trophozoite next to the nucleus. Four flagella are present; three of them extend anteriorly at the broad end of the trophozoite, while one extends posteriorly from the cytostome. A spiral groove extends across the ventral surface, resulting in a curved appearance at the posterior end.

   When seen in wet preparations, the trophozoite of *G. lamblia* shows an erratic type of motility described as being like a "falling leaf," while that of *C. mesnili* exhibits a stiff, rotary directional type of motility. However, since most fecal specimens are received in preservatives, it is usually impossible to determine this characteristic.

3. Although *C. mesnili* is not considered to be pathogenic for humans, the presence of this parasite in a patient's stool specimen indicates previous ingestion of food or water contaminated by an individual infected with this ameba.

4. The cyst stage of *C. mesnili* is pear shaped and ranges from 6 to 10 μm long, and from 4 to 6 μm wide. The cyst contains a single nucleus, with the chromatin often condensed, appearing as a large, central karyosome. A prominent, curved cytostomal fibril known as a "shepherd's crook" may also be visible. Each cyst is characterized by the presence of a protuberance or nipple, giving it the appearance of a lemon. This characteristic is not found in any of the other intestinal protozoan parasites.

A 19-year-old female university student reported to the college infirmary, with complaints of diarrhea, nausea, and vomiting. A physician ordered stool specimens to be sent to the infirmary laboratory for examination for ova and parasites. The permanent trichrome stain revealed a moderate number of ameboid trophozoites, with finely granular cytoplasm and evenly distributed peripheral nuclear chromatin. No ingested red blood cells were seen. A characteristic trophozoite is shown in Fig. 60.1. No cyst forms were observed.

The medical technologist consulted pictures in a textbook and found morphologic similarities of the trophozoites to those of the *Entamoeba histolytica/Entamoeba dispar* group. The pathogenic *E. histolytica* causes amebic dysentery. However, on careful examination of the trichrome-stained smear using a calibrated ocular micrometer, the technologist measured the trophozoites at 5 to 12 μm in diameter.

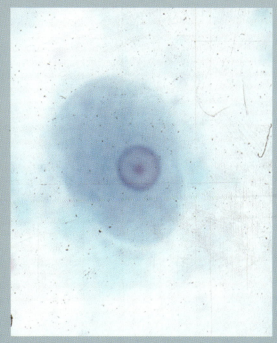

Figure 60.1

QUESTIONS

1. Which parasite was probably seen by the medical technologist?

2. Discuss the importance of using a calibrated ocular micrometer to identify parasites.

3. Other than intestinal parasites, which other infectious agents might be causing this patient's symptoms? How would this diagnosis be made?

4. How is the diagnosis of amebic dysentery made in the laboratory?

5. Describe the life cycle of this parasite.

6. How is infection with this parasite transmitted?

7. How can the spread of this infection be prevented?

ANSWERS

1. The trophozoites seen by the medical technologist in the trichrome stained smear measured 5 to 12 μm and were probably trophozoites of *Entamoeba hartmanni,* which is not known to be pathogenic in humans. They were too small to be those of the *E. histolytica/E. dispar* group, which measure 12 to 60 μm. *E. hartmanni* was formerly known as "small-race *E. histolytica*" due to its small size and morphological similarity to that ameba.

2. To ensure the accurate identification of parasites, especially amebic trophozoites and cysts, it is essential to carefully measure them with an ocular micrometer. An ocular micrometer may be calibrated by using a calibrated objective micrometer. The ocular micrometer must be recalibrated for each objective and microscope used. This should allow any medical technologist to distinguish between *E. hartmanni* and *E. histolytica/E. dispar.*

3. The patient might be infected with pathogenic bacilli, such as *Shigella, Salmonella,* or *Campylobacter* species. These enteric bacilli may be isolated when a routine bacterial culture of a stool specimen is ordered. Cultures for *Yersinia* and *Vibrio* species, which are also enteric pathogens, are usually performed on request, based on clinical findings. Viruses may also cause similar symptoms. Viral cultures and enzyme immunoassays for selected agents are also generally available.

4. The laboratory diagnosis of amebic dysentery is usually made by examination of fecal specimens for the presence of typical trophozoites and cysts of *E. histolytica.* Successful diagnosis is dependent on collection of proper specimens and examination by well-trained and experienced laboratory personnel. Direct saline wet preparations may be useful in detecting motile trophozoites, especially in fresh liquid stool specimens. These examinations are usually not possible, however, since most fecal specimens are collected in preservatives.

   Concentration techniques may allow the observation of amebic cysts. However, the permanent stained smear, such as the trichrome or iron hematoxylin stain, is most useful in the identification of amebic trophozoites and cysts. A permanent stained smear should be made for all stool specimens, regardless of the consistency of the specimen. A minimum of three specimens should be collected over 10 days. Microscopic methods do not usually allow differentiation of the pathogenic species *E. histolytica* from the nonpathogenic species *E. dispar.*

   Antigen detection methods have been successful in diagnosing amebiasis. Immunofluorescent-antibody methods and enzyme immunoassays have been developed for the detection of the *E. histolytica/E. dispar* antigen in stool specimens. Some of these tests have shown sensitivities and specificities comparable to or better than those of microscopic examination for cysts or trophozoites.

   In addition to a microtiter format, immunochromatographic lateral-flow membrane assays, using a cartridge format, are available and provide sensitive, specific, rapid, and easy-to-read immunoassays for the diagnosis of amebiasis. This method relies on capillary action, since parasite antigens are captured by a specific antibody as the sample moves laterally through the unit. These kits may have limited use, however, since fresh or frozen stool is required and most fecal specimens are collected in preservatives. Although most of these assays are unable to distinguish the pathogenic *E. histolytica* from the nonpathogenic *E. dispar,* one commercially available kit can do so. If differentiation between *E. histolytica* and *E. dispar* is needed, a fresh unfixed specimen should be requested.

5. Infection with *E. hartmanni* begins when mature cysts (the infective stage) are ingested. The mature cyst passes through the stomach and excysts in the lower ileum of the small intestine. Here the cyst develops into the trophozoite form and multiplies by binary fission. Trophozoites continue to reproduce in the lumen of the colon, where they may encyst. Immature cysts (with one or two nuclei) are passed in the feces, although cysts may develop to maturity (with four nuclei) before being excreted. Trophozoites, immature cysts, and mature cysts may be found in the feces, although trophozoites are usually found only in liquid feces.

6. Transmission of intestinal amebae, including *E. hartmanni,* usually occurs by the fecal-oral route, whereby water contaminated with amebic cysts is ingested.

7. Transmission could be prevented by good personal hygiene and improvement in sanitary practices.

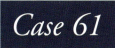

Case 61

A 43-year-old man, who had been hospitalized for 2 weeks in the intensive care unit for pneumonia, was released in apparently good health. He had been treated with a number of antibiotics, including clindamycin, for his pneumonia. A few days later, he returned to the emergency department complaining of crampy abdominal pain, malaise, nausea, fever and bloody diarrhea. He had been passing 8 to 10 loose stools daily.

Stool specimens were sent to the laboratory for routine cultures for enteric bacterial pathogens and examination for ova and parasites. Stool cultures were negative for bacterial pathogens, and no ova and parasites were seen on any microscopic examinations of the specimens. Over the next few days, his symptoms worsened, and he was readmitted to the hospital.

QUESTIONS

1. Since routine cultures for bacterial pathogens were negative and no parasites were detected, which other bacterial infection might explain the patient's symptoms?

2. Why would this bacterium not have been identified in the routine culture for bacterial pathogens?

3. How does this infection develop?

4. How is this infection treated?

5. Which laboratory tests are available to diagnose this infection?

ANSWERS

1. The patient's history is notable for his hospitalization in the intensive care unit for pneumonia. The patient most probably had been treated with large doses of antibiotics, which would predispose him to infection with *Clostridium difficile*. The patient might be suffering from antibiotic-associated diarrhea or the more serious pseudomembranous colitis caused by this anaerobic bacterium.

2. This bacterium is not usually identified when a routine culture for enteric pathogens is ordered. Routine cultures for enteric bacterial pathogens usually include media to rule out *Salmonella, Shigella,* and *Campylobacter.* Media may be added to detect other pathogens, including diarrheagenic *Escherichia coli* and *Vibrio* species.

3. The prolonged use of antibiotics, especially in patients in hospitals and nursing homes, alters the suppressive activity of the normal intestinal flora and allows the overgrowth of *C. difficile.* Clindamycin has long been associated with this infection. The toxins of *C. difficile* damage the colonic mucosa, leading to diarrhea, colitis, and possible colonic perforation. Toxic megacolon may occur when the disease is particularly severe. The colitis associated with *C. difficile* diarrhea most often affects the entire colon, although left-sided colitis is more common than right-sided colitis.

4. Antimicrobial agents used to treat infections with *C. difficile* include metronidazole and vancomycin.

5. The laboratory diagnosis of infection with *C. difficile* may be made in several ways. The microorganism may be grown in culture by using specially formulated media, such as CCFA (cycloserine-cefoxitin-fructose-egg yolk agar). Cultures are expensive and time-consuming and are usually used only in the epidemiological investigation of outbreaks and selected clinical situations. *C. difficile* received its name because it is difficult to grow in culture. If the microorganism is grown in culture, toxigenicity should be confirmed by cell culture, since not all strains of *C. difficile* produce toxins. *C. difficile* diarrhea is a result of toxin-mediated inflammation. Nontoxigenic strains of *C. difficile* may be present in healthy adults.

Two toxins are produced by *C. difficile.* Toxin A is an enterotoxin which increases intestinal permeability and leads to enteric fluid collection and diarrhea. Toxin B is a cytotoxin which causes cytopathic effects in several tissue culture lines but whose actions in vivo are not completely understood. Toxin B may act synergistically with toxin A. Two types of tests are available for the detection of toxin. Tissue culture remains the "gold standard" for the detection of the cytotoxin (toxin B), because of its sensitivity and specificity. This assay is laborious and slow, requiring 48 h of incubation, and is not practical for routine clinical use.

Rapid enzyme immunoassays are commercially available for the detection of toxin A; combination assays are available to detect toxins A and B. Although most strains of *C. difficile* produce both toxins A and B or neither, strains that are toxin A negative and toxin B positive have recently been isolated from clinical specimens.

A latex agglutination assay exists for the detection of glutamate dehydrogenase, a clostridial enzyme. PCR assays for bacterial DNA amplification are currently being investigated. Colonoscopy may be used to establish a diagnosis by allowing the visualization of plaques or pseudomembranes on the mucous membranes of the colon.

Case 62

In January, a previously healthy 3-year-old girl presented to the emergency department with symptoms of fever, diarrhea, and vomiting of several days' duration. She was dehydrated but otherwise in good health.

A stool specimen was submitted to the laboratory for bacterial culture and an examination for ova and parasites. No enteric pathogens were isolated from culture. Concentration procedures were performed, and a permanent smear using the trichrome stain was prepared. Microscopic examination of the trichrome stain revealed a few trophozoites (measuring 6 to 12 μm) of an ameba, which was identified as *Endolimax nana*. The nuclear membrane of these trophozoites lacked peripheral nuclear chromatin. The cytoplasm was finely vacuolated. A large, central, dotlike karyosome was evident in the nucleus. Figure 62.1 shows the trophozoite form of this parasite. Several cyst forms, measuring 5 to 10 μm and containing four nuclei with blotlike karyosomes, were also seen in the smear.

The patient was treated for this amebic parasite with metronidazole and made an uneventful recovery following oral rehydration therapy.

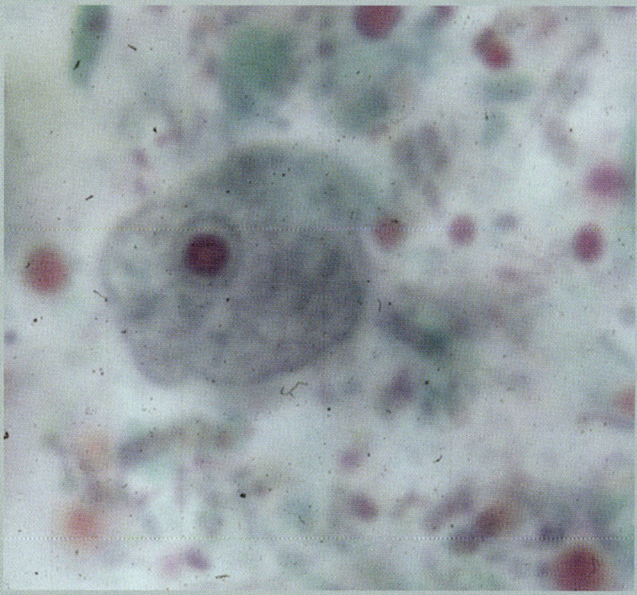

Figure 62.1

QUESTIONS

1. Was this patient treated appropriately? Explain. Is metronidazole an appropriate therapy for any amebic infection?

2. What is the probable cause of this child's symptoms? Is this infection associated with a seasonal occurrence?

3. How would you diagnose this infection?

4. Describe the life cycle of this parasite.

5. How did this child probably acquire this infection?

6. How would you microscopically distinguish the pathogen *Entamoeba histolytica* from *E. nana*?

7. List other amebae which must be morphologically distinguished from the previous two parasites when identified in a stool specimen.

ANSWERS

1. The patient should not have been treated with metronidazole. *E. nana* is non-pathogenic and does not require treatment. The pathogenic ameba *Entamoeba histolytica* should be treated, either with metronidazole or with another amebicidal agent such as iodoquinol or diloxanide furoate.

2. The differential diagnosis of diarrheal infections in children includes bacterial infection, intestinal parasites, and viruses. There was no evidence of the presence of bacterial or parasitic pathogens in the stool specimen submitted for laboratory analysis.

   Viral gastroenteritis is second only to viral respiratory disease in the United States. No tests for viruses were performed on the child's stool specimen. Although several viruses, including rotaviruses, enteric adenoviruses, astroviruses, and noroviruses, may cause gastroenteritis, rotaviruses are the most common cause of this illness in young children. This patient was likely suffering from gastroenteritis due to rotavirus infection. Vomiting and dehydration are common symptoms of gastroenteritis caused by the rotaviruses. This fact, together with the seasonality (rotavirus infections are more common in the winter months) has led to the term "winter vomiting disease." The association of vomiting with this infection may be related to the age of the patient rather than the nature of the virus.

3. Rotaviruses, due to their fastidious nature, are not readily grown in culture. The laboratory diagnosis of rotavirus infection is usually made by the direct detection of viral antigen, using one of the available enzyme-linked immunosorbent assays or latex agglutination tests. The use of monoclonal antibodies has increased the sensitivity and specificity of these assays, although a high rate of false-positive reactions has occurred with neonates.

4. The infection begins when mature cysts (the infective stage) are ingested. The mature cyst passes through the stomach and excysts in the lower ileum of the small intestine, where the cyst develops into the trophozoite form and multiplies by binary fission. Trophozoites continue to multiply in the lumen of the colon and may become encysted. Immature cysts are rarely passed in the feces. Trophozoites and mature cysts may be found in the stool specimen.

5. Amebic infections are transmitted mostly by the ingestion of fecally contaminated food and water which contain amebic cysts. After ingestion, excystation occurs. Asymptomatic carriers are important in the transmission and spread of disease, since they generally harbor only cysts, which are more resistant to environmental effects than are trophozoites. The infection is easily spread among children in a nursery setting, since they are in such close contact with each other.

6. The trophozoite form of *Entamoeba histolytica* measures 12 to 60 μm and has evenly distributed peripheral nuclear chromatin. The compact karyosome is small and central. The trophozoite of *E. nana* measures 6 to 12 μm and lacks peripheral nuclear chromatin. This amebic parasite has a large, central or eccentric, dotlike karyosome. The mature cyst of *Entamoeba histolytica* measures 10 to 20 μm and

has elongated chromatoidal bars with rounded, blunt, smooth ends. The cysts of *Endolimax nana* measure 5 to 10 μm and lack chromatoid bars.

7. Other intestinal amebae which must be distinguished from *Entamoeba histolytica* and *E. nana* include *Entamoeba dispar, Entamoeba hartmanni, Entamoeba coli, Entamoeba polecki,* and *Iodamoeba bütschlii.*

REFERENCES

Ash, L. R., and T. C. Orihel. 1991. *Parasites: a Guide to Laboratory Procedures and Identification.* ASCP Press, Chicago, Ill.

Centers for Disease Control and Prevention. 2002. Norwalk-like virus-associated gastroenteritis in a large, high-density encampment—Virginia, July 2001. *Morb. Mortal. Wkly. Rep.* **51:**661–663.

Clark, C. G., and L. S. Diamond. 2002. Methods for cultivation of luminal parasitic protists of clinical importance. *Clin. Microbiol. Rev.* **15:**329–341.

Garcia, L. S. 2001. *Diagnostic Medical Parasitology,* 4th ed. ASM Press, Washington, D.C.

Heelan, J. S., and F. W. Ingersoll. 2002. *Essentials of Human Parasitology.* Thomson Delmar Learning, Albany, N.Y.

Koneman, E. W., S. D. Allen, W. M. Janda, P. C. Schreckenberger, and W. C. Winn, Jr. 1997. *Color Atlas and Textbook of Diagnostic Microbiology,* 5th ed. Lippincott Publications, Philadelphia, Pa.

Leber, A. L., and S. M. Novak. 1999. Intestinal and urogenital amebae, flagellates, and ciliates, p. 1391–1405. *In* P. R. Murray, E. J. Baron, M. A. Pfaller, F. C. Tenover, and R. H. Yolken (ed.), *Manual of Clinical Microbiology,* 7th ed. ASM Press, Washington, D.C.

Lyerly, D. M., H. C. Krivan, and T. D. Wilkins. 1988. *Clostridium difficile:* its disease and toxins. *Clin. Microbiol. Rev.* **1:**1–18.

Markell, E. K., D. T. John, and W. A. Krotoski. 1999. *Markell and Voge's Medical Parasitology,* 8th ed. The W. B. Saunders Co., Philadelphia, Pa.

Mirelman, D. 1987. Effect of culture conditions and bacterial associates on the zymodemes of *Entamoeba histolytica. Parasitol Today* **3:**37–40.

Shimeld, L., and A. T. Rodgers. 1999. Intestinal and atrial protozoans, p. 572–589. *In* L. Shimeld, (ed.), *Essentials of Diagnostic Microbiology.* Thomson Delmar Learning, Albany, N.Y.

Zaki, M., P. Meelu, W. Sun, and C. G. Clark. 2002. Simultaneous differentiation and typing of *Entamoeba histolytica* and *Entamoeba dispar. J. Clin. Microbiol.* **40:**1271–1276.

Zeibig, E. A. 1997. *Clinical Parasitology,* p. 37–60. The W. B. Saunders Co., Philadelphia, Pa.

Glossary

Acanthopodia Spiky projections present on the pseudopods of *Acanthamoeba* trophozoites.

Accolé forms *See* Appliqué forms.

Amastigotes Intracellular developmental stages in the life cycle of *Leishmania* species and *Trypanosoma cruzi*.

Anorexia Lack of appetite.

Appliqué forms Early-ring-stage trophozoites of *Plasmodium falciparum*, found at the periphery of red blood cells. Also called accolé forms.

Axoneme The intracellular portion of a flagellum.

Axostyle A rodlike structure running the length of a flagellate, which provides rigidity to the parasite.

Bancroftian filariasis Lymphatic filariasis caused by *Wuchereria bancrofti*.

Benign tertian malaria Malaria caused by *Plasmodium vivax*.

Binary fission Multiplication of a cell by splitting into two equal daughter cells.

Blackwater fever A rare complication of malaria, usually *Plasmodium falciparum* malaria. Massive intravascular hemolysis causes hemoglobinuria, with a blackening of the urine, due to a high methemoglobin level in the urine.

Bothria Shallow longitudinal sucking grooves found on the scolex of the broad (or fish) tapeworm *Diphyllobothrium latum*.

Bradyzoite A slowly multiplying trophozoite stage in the life cycle of *Toxoplasma gondii*.

Calabar (fugitive) swellings Localized patches of subcutaneous edema seen in individuals infected with the African eye worm, *Loa loa*.

Central-body form One form of *Blastocystis hominis*, characterized by a large, transparent vacuole.

Cercaria A free-living larva of a trematode (fluke).

Cestode A tapeworm.

Chagoma A painful, erythematous, indurated local lesion which may develop at the site of inoculation of trypomastigotes of *Trypanosoma cruzi*.

Chiclero ulcer Common name for New World cutaneous leishmaniasis in Mexico, caused by a hemoflagellate in the *Leishmania mexicana* complex.

Chromatin DNA; peripheral nuclear chromatin is found in members of the *Entamoeba* genus of protozoans.

Chromatoid body A darkly stained round or rod-shaped structure consisting of DNA found in certain amebic cysts. Also called chromatoid bar.

Cilia Short, numerous organelles of locomotion found in protozoan ciliates.

Copepod A small crustacean which serves as an intermediate host for certain parasites.

Coracidium A ciliated larval tapeworm which develops in the eggs of *Diphyllobothrium latum*.

Cribriform plate The sievelike portion of the ethmoid bone.

Cutaneous Relating to the skin.

Cutaneous larva migrans Migration of larvae through skin.

Cyst An inactive, dormant, resistant protozoan form.

Cysticercoids Larvae of *Dipylidium caninum* and *Hymenolepis* species.

Cysticercus The larval stage of the pork and beef tapeworms *Taenia solium* and *T. saginata*. It has a single scolex invaginated into a fluid-filled cyst.

Cytopyge An excretory pore found in certain protozoa.

Cytostome An oral groove found in certain protozoa.

Decorticated Lacking the mammillated outer covering; used to describe eggs of *Ascaris lumbricoides*.

Definitive host The host in which sexual reproduction of a parasite takes place.

Diurnal Daylight related.

Dyspnea Difficulty in breathing.

Embryonated Containing an embryo.

Eosinophilia A state characterized by a large number of eosinophils; often associated with helminth infections.

Espundia The name given to mucocutaneous leishmaniasis in Brazil.

Filariform larva The infective third-stage larva of the hookworm and *Strongyloides stercoralis*.

Flagella Long, whiplike organelles of locomotion found in flagellates.

Fluke A trematode.

Fomite An inanimate object.

Free-living protozoa Parasites which inhabit bodies of soil and water.

Gametocyte A sex (male or female) cell of a malaria parasite.

Gravid Full of eggs.

Halzoun An uncommon syndrome, once thought to be caused by the attachment of adult worms or larvae of *Fasciola hepatica* to the pharyngeal mucosa, resulting in edema and congestion of the soft palate, which may result in pain, dyspnea, dysphagia, and, occasionally, suffocation. It is now thought to be caused by nymphs of pentastomes (linguatulids), which are wormlike parasites inhabiting the respiratory passages of carnivorous reptiles, birds, and mammals.

Helminth A worm that may be a nematode (roundworm), cestode (tapeworm), or trematode (fluke).

Hematuria The presence of blood or hemoglobin in the urine.

Hemozoin A pigment found in erythrocytes in malarial infection but not in cases of babesiosis.

Hydatid cyst A cyst that develops as a result of infection with *Echinococcus granulosus*. The cyst has a thick, laminated outer layer and an inner layer of germinal epithelial tissue from which the daughter cysts and brood capsules (smaller cysts containing several developing inverted scolices) bud into the cavity of the cyst.

Hydatid sand Granular material consisting of free scolices, free cysts, and amorphous germinal material of *Echinococcus granulosus*.

Hypnozoites Resting sporozoites found in infections with *Plasmodium vivax* and *Plasmodium ovale*. When reactivated, they are responsible for relapses common in these infections.

Intermediate host A host in which larval development occurs in the developmental cycle of certain parasites.

Kala-azar Old World visceral leishmaniasis caused by a member of the *Leishmania donovani* complex.

Karyosome A clump of chromatin in the nucleus of amebae. The shape, size, and location of the karyosome are characteristic for different amebae and are used in the identification of these parasites.

Kerandel's sign The delayed sensation of pain in patients with African trypanosomiasis.

Keratitis Corneal inflammation.

Kissing bug The common name for the reduviid or triatomid bug, the vector for *Trypanosoma cruzi*.

Leishmanoid A condition characterized by the development of erythematous or depigmented macules, which may occur after treatment for visceral leishmaniasis.

Leukocytosis A high white blood cell count.

Macrogamete A female sex cell.

Malignant tertian malaria *Plasmodium falciparum* malaria.

Maltese cross A tetrad formation of chromatin found in erythrocytes in patients with babesiosis.

Mammillated Covered with an albuminous outer covering usually present on the eggs of the roundworm, *Ascaris lumbricoides*.

Maurer's dots Dots found in red blood cells, characteristic of infection with *Plasmodium falciparum*.

Median bodies Structures, found in *Giardia lamblia,* which cross the axonemes at an angle which results in the appearance of a mouth. Also called parabasal bodies.

Merogony Schizogony or fission.

Merozoite A segment of a malarial schizont.

Metacercariae Encysted cercariae of intestinal trematodes. They are found in the flesh of vertebrates and invertebrates, as well as on freshwater vegetation.

Microfilariae Wormlike larvae produced by nematodes called filariae.

Microgamete A male sex cell.

Miracidium A larva of a trematode (fluke).

Nematode A roundworm.

Neural larva migrans Migration of the larvae of animal nematodes through the human central nervous system.

Nocturnal Night related.

Ocular larva migrans Migration of the larvae of animal nematodes through the human eye.

Ocular micrometer A measuring device used to determine the size of objects observed under a microscope.

Onchocercomas Subcutaneous painless nodules which contain adult worms and are found on the skin of patients infected with *Onchocerca volvulus*.

Oncosphere The six-hooked embryo of a tapeworm.

Oocyst The developmental structure of coccidian protozoan parasites.

Ookinete A structure that develops when a *Plasmodium* zygote puts out a pseudopod, which becomes elongated. The motile ookinete develops into a spherical oocyst in the gut wall of a mosquito.

Operculum An opening in a helminth eggshell which acts as an "escape hatch" for the embryo.

Oriental sore Old World cutaneous leishmaniasis.

Parabasal bodies *See* Median bodies.

Parasite An organism living in or on another organism and being dependent on this organism, known as the host.

Plerocercoid larva An infective larva of *Diphyllobothrium latum,* which develops in the flesh of the freshwater fish, the second intermediate host.

Polar filaments Filaments that arise from polar thickenings on the embryo wall of the smallest human tapeworm, *Hymenolepis nana*. *See also* Polar tubule.

Polar tubule An extrusion mechanism found in microsporidian protozoans. Also called polar filament.

Procercoid larva A larva which develops in a copepod, the first intermediate host for the tapeworm *Diphyllobothrium latum*.

Proglottid A segment of the strobila of a tapeworm.

Promastigote An elongated, motile, infective form of a hemoflagellate.

Pseudomembranous colitis Gastrointestinal illness caused by the bacterium *Clostridium difficile*, usually following a prolonged course of antimicrobial therapy.

Pseudopod Extension of cytoplasm which serves as an organelle of locomotion found in amebae.

Quartan malaria Malaria characterized by a 72-h periodicity, associated with infections caused by *Plasmodium malariae*.

Rediae Developmental stages of trematodes which may develop into daughter rediae or cercariae.

Reduviid bug A vector for *Trypanosoma cruzi*.

Reticulocyte A young red blood cell.

Rhabditiform larva A free-living, noninfective first-stage larva of the hookworm and *Strongyloides stercoralis*.

Romaña's sign Unilateral edema affecting the eyelids, which occurs in infections with *Trypanosoma cruzi*.

Rostellum A crown-shaped structure found on the scolex of a tapeworm to which hooklets are usually attached.

Schistosomulum A stage that forms after the free-swimming cercariae of *Schistosoma mansoni* enter the host by penetrating human skin.

Schizogony A form of asexual reproduction of the malarial parasites, which occurs within red blood cells.

Schüffner's dots Eosinophilic stippling found in erythrocytes infected with *Plasmodium vivax* and *Plasmodium ovale*.

Scolex The anterior part of a tapeworm which may bear suckers, grooves, or a rostellum with hooks, depending on the species, and which is responsible for attachment to the intestinal mucosa.

Sheath The outer covering of the microfilariae of some species of filarial nematodes.

Sporocyst Stage that forms after a trematode miracidium infects a snail; forms during the developmental cycle of certain sporozoa.

Sporogony Spore production in the microsporidia; sexual reproduction of malarial parasites in the mosquito, with the production of sporozoites.

Sporozoite Infective stage of the malarial parasites, which is inoculated into humans when bitten by a mosquito.

Steatorrhea Presence of fat in the stool as a result of malabsorption.

Sucking disk The area that covers the ventral side of *Giardia lamblia*. It provides a mechanism by which the parasite attaches to the mucosa of the small intestine.

Swimmer's itch Dermatitis caused when the cercariae of bird schistosomes penetrate human skin.

Tachyzoite An actively multiplying developmental stage in the life cycle of certain protozoa such as *Toxoplasma gondii*.

Tapeworm A cestode; composed of a scolex, a neck, where growth occurs, and a chain of proglottids known as a strobila.

Tertian malaria Malaria characterized by a 48-h periodicity, associated with infections caused by *Plasmodium falciparum*, *Plasmodium vivax*, and *Plasmodium ovale*.

Trematode A helminth known as a fluke.

Triatomid bug A vector of Chagas' disease.

Trophozoite Motile, actively reproducing form of protozoa.

Trypomastigote Trypanosome stage found in human blood in the life cycle of trypanosomes.

Visceral larva migrans Migration of the larvae of animal nematodes through the viscera.

Whipworm The common name for the nematode *Trichuris trichiura*.

Winterbottom's sign Enlargement of lymph nodes in the posterior cervical region in patients with African trypanosomiasis.

Zoonosis An infection acquired from animals.

Zygote Fertilized stage resulting from the union of male and female gametes.

List of Figures

SECTION III   CESTODES, TREMATODES, AND INTESTINAL NEMATODES

SECTION IV BLOOD AND TISSUE NEMATODES

SECTION V CHALLENGING CASES

Index

Note: Page references in italics denote figures.

Trophozoites, *see* specific parasites
Trypanosoma brucei gambiense, 53, 59, 59–61, 88
Trypanosoma brucei rhodesiense, 53, 60–61, 87, 87–88
Trypanosoma cruzi, 53, 61, 93, 93–95
Tsetse fly, 53, 60, 87–88

V

Vancomycin, for *Clostridium difficile*, 222
Vittaforma corneae, 44

W

Whipworm, *see Trichuris trichiura*
Wuchereria bancrofti, 171, *181*, 181–183, 186

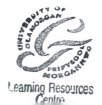